The Year of Shaving Dangerously:

Dispatches from the Front Lines of Manliness

M. Blake Roberts

To Amanda,

who lovingly accepted and

encouraged my new found hobby,

even when I had much more

important things to do.

<u>Special Thanks</u>

This never would have happened without the encouragement of many friends and strangers, of which a few stand out:

Colin Reid, for first informing me that double-edge razors exist.

Ronald Swart, for his extensive advice and for volunteering to edit a book about shaving. Of all the ways you could have used your time, thank you for spending some of it on me.

The internet, where I learned so much. Of special note are the forums We the Armed, and Arizona Gun Owners, as well as the websites Shaving 101, Sharpologist, Shaveology, and Leisure Guy.

The folks of Criterion Journal (and others). You know who you are.

And most importantly, my family. Mom and Dad, thank you for not leaving me to the wolves, even when I gave you early grey hair. I can never repay how much you've done for me. Amanda, thank you for all the love, support, editing, and willingness to part with our monies in pursuit of my hobby. You're the best!

Cover art and design by:

Forty {3} Graphic Marketing

Manifest

The Beginning

In November of 2013 I bought my first double-edge (DE) safety razor.

Unlike cartridge razors, which are intended to only use one of a couple blade types designed by whichever company made the handle, DE razors accept blades that might come from any of dozens of manufacturers. Some of those blades are new, some have been around for decades, and different blades will give you a different shaving experience.

I grew up shaving with a Mach 3, and so this was a whole new world to me. I'd never had to worry about what type of blade I was getting, what the differences were, or finding the right combination of blade and razor to fit my face. The handle went into the cartridge, and that was it. Cuts were virtually non-existent, and I almost never even bothered with shaving cream, much less aftershave or any other shave treatments. Shaving was because I had to (either for work, school, or some other reason), that was it.

At the recommendation of a friend who was already into DE shaving, after a month or so of figuring things out I picked up a razor blade sampler pack. Since there are so many type of blades out there, sampler packs allow you to try just a few blades of a collection of brands so you can figure out what works best for you. For a newcomer like me this was ideal, as I had almost no idea what brands even existed, much less which ones were good.

So for $15 I got a pack that included 46 blades from eight different brands, and last week I began my attempt to work my way through them. With each blade lasting a week (they could be pushed to last longer without much problem, but a week seems like a good standard to go by), it'll take me months to complete.

I'm figuring this out as I go, so we'll see what happens along the way.

My starting tools:

Edwin Jagger De89L razor, Col. Conk shaving soap, badger hair brush, and razor sampler pack, purchased from bullgooseshaving.com.

Let the journey begin!

Cream of the Crop

January 14, 2014

Monday was a banner day in my quest to relearn shaving: for the first time since I started doing home mixed, brush and lather shaving, I managed to make a foam that was pretty much perfect. Not too wet, not too dry, just rich, silky, and foamy.

I was so happy I ran into the other room to show Amanda. And by show, I mean smear some on her while she was doing her makeup (just on her hand though, I'm not a jerk).

Shaving cream and I don't have a long history together. I figured out about ten years ago that I really didn't need it. I didn't feel a lot different, it's about impossible to cut yourself whether you use it or not, and it costs money. I pretty much never got razor burn, so a splash of water on my face would be the most I used unless for some reason somebody gave me a can.

That changed with DE shaving. Technically, I don't know how it would go if I tried doing it with just water, as I've not tried it. As I get more comfortable shaving this way I might give it a try just to see what happens, and if I cut my lips off or something I'll be sure to write about it for the amusement of the world.

In the meanwhile, I'm rediscovering shaving cream. Shortly after I got my razor I picked up a tiny travel can of Barbasol and that lasted me a few weeks. It wasn't terrible by any means, and I didn't feel a strong need to use anything else.

But with friends singing the praises of home lathering, and Amanda looking for a Christmas gift for me, it seemed like a good time to try it out. I got a badger hair brush and a bar of actual shaving soap, and for the last ten days I've been trying it out.

I don't know if it actually makes for a better shave in the sense of better skin, or cleaner cuts. And I wouldn't say that it is as big of an improvement as DE shaving was over cartridges. But, it absolutely makes for a better shave experience.

First, it just smells better. My current soap is Bayrum, and man does it smell nice. Just this morning my wife announced during breakfast "you smell manly." Can't go wrong with that, and since I've started the bathroom where I shave has developed a nice smell all day long. Second, there's something to be said to building a new skill and seeing results. My first attempts were, to be mild, not great. Now, while I'm still building the skill, I'm starting to see some good results and that's making me want to be better. And third, it does feel better. Cream from a can is fine, but home lather has a nice warmth to it, and seems to just sit a bit better on the face. Is it a huge difference? No, but it's noticeable.

Parallel to my razor blade test, I'll also be trying out different lathers. The CVS by my house sells a few simple shaving soaps and powders, which are dirt cheap compared to a lot of what's out there. I expect

4

that you get what you pay for, but I'll give it a try and see how it works. Might as well, if it's cheap and it works great then it's attractive to me.

One Pass, Two Pass, Red Pass, Smooth Pass

January 16, 2014

I shave against the grain, a habit that's probably going to get me in trouble one day. Every shave blog and traditional wet shaving instructional I've seen tells beginners not to do it, but each morning I find myself with an upside down razor merrily clear cutting the black forest.

So far I've managed to get away with it, I've only nicked myself once and that wasn't really an issue of against the grain but rather getting quick and sloppy. I almost never get razor burn or ingrown hairs, so that's not really a concern either. The worst I've gotten is a spot of blood here or there, which washes off and closes up with a good cold water rinse and aftershave. Instead, I've found that going against the grain from the start has several advantages for me:

First, it's more satisfying when I'm shaving. You feel the slightest bit of resistance, which suddenly gives way when the razor is angled just right…
magical. Going with the grain feels smooth, but this feels like it's getting something done.

Second, it saves time. My wife leaves for work before I do, and I generally make breakfast so she can get out the door with less stress and rush. Going against the grain allows for a close, consistent shave with just one pass. While I'm enjoying shaving as a process and experience, I do have day to day time constraints to deal with.

Today though I decided to do a couple things different. First, I decided to try applying the lather in a "paint brush" stroke rather than circular (I'll talk about this more in detail another time, simply out though: it feels wonderful). Second, I decided to try doing the "beard reduction" method of at least one pass with the grain before lathering again and going against.

It probably only took an extra few minutes, but I've got to admit that the results feel pretty good.

I don't know that it's that much closer. If anything, it might not feel quite as slick when I run my hand with the grain. But, when I run my hand against the grain it feels noticeably better. With one pass there will be an occasional scratchy/ sharp hair that's only really noticeable when I'm checking against the grain. This time, while it doesn't feel quite as close, it feels more even with no sharpness. And not a spot of bleeding, that's a plus.

I don't know that I'll do this every time, but it's something I'm going to keep working on. When I get to the really sharp blades, like the Feather, it might be good to be used to doing more passes rather than a one swipe wonder. I'd really rather not cut my face off, as that would put a real damper on the day. What I want to find out is whether with more time, attention, and practice this will result in a uniform shave that is close, smooth, and worth the extra time and effort.

Review: Shark Super Stainless

January 17, 2014

As part of the ongoing experiment, for the last two weeks I've been trying out Shark Super Stainless razor blades. Made in Egypt, the blades lacked the numbering system that I had gotten used to and so I was pretty much just winging it on which side of the razor to use each day. (Many double-edge (DE) razor blades have numbers printed on the razor, which I understand to be something that happens during quality control, and which some people use to keep track of which sides of the razor they recently used.)

Before I get into the Shark blades, a quick word on Derby razor blades. When I purchased my razor it came with a pack of Derby blades, which I thought did a great job. In fact, I considered just not bothering to see what other blades were out there because I was perfectly satisfied with the shave that they gave me. While I don't have a scientific measuring system for my tests, I'll probably refer back to Derby from time to time as they are what I'm using as a rough benchmark for performance. Now, on to the review…

I am very satisfied with the Shark blade. All of my shaves during the first week, from Monday to Friday, were some of the best shaves I've had with my razor thus far (several were easily the best shaves I've ever had at home). The shaves have been smooth, extremely close, and yet have given me less irritation than I've seem to have gotten from the Derby blades.

I suspect this might be because the blade is sharper (it feels like it is), and so it can shave closer with less tugging and irritation. Only one nick, the first I've had yet, and it was so minor that it was completely resolved with cold water and aftershave.

This week saw even more improvement. Combining with better skill at lathering, and improved technique and practice at shaving, the last two days are probably my two best shaves since I've started shaving. I wrote yesterday about one, and today has been even better (far and away better, today's shave really nailed it).

The experiment is just starting, but already I think it's safe to say I'm not going back to Derby blades. While I have no complaints about Derby, Shark seems to have outperformed them where it counts: on my face. I'm glad I've got three more of their blades to enjoy.

I intend to hold on to them and start using a new brand next week. Later in the year I'll come back to the Sharks and see how they stack up against the wider field of competition.

Shave on!

<u>Why am I Shaving Like This?</u>

January 19, 2014

The first two questions I usually get when someone finds out I'm trying out traditional wet shaving are usually some form of "what is a double edge razor" and "why would you use one?" There are a lot of lists out there giving reasons to do it (less irritation, less ingrown hairs, etc.). Here's my story:

I knew about straight razor shaving, but aside from that I was neither aware nor concerned about other types of shaving out there until around the last year or so. My first hint was when a shooting buddy of mine mentioned on an internet forum that he used a double edge safety razor, which I'd never heard of before. Like any inquisitive person my age, I googled it.

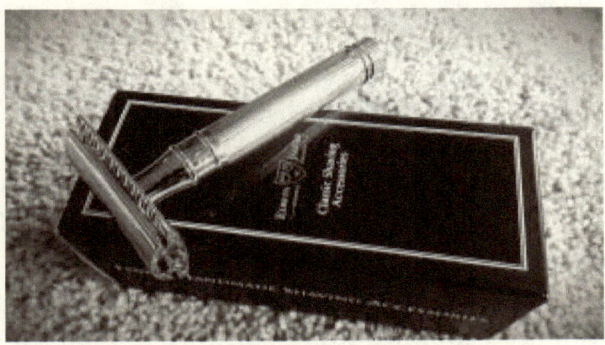

A modern, double-edge safety razor. (comma after modern)

While safety razors (called such because it offered some protection from the blade unlike open straight razors) date back to the mid 1800's, the double edge safety razor originated in 1903 when King (name, not title) Gillette patented the first design for one. Selling just a few dozen his first year, within three years his company would be selling more than 300,000.

The advantages were simple: it was harder to cut yourself, the blades were easy to replace and had no need of sharpening, and the double edge meant that you could shave twice as often between changing blades. Less work, more safety, more bang for your buck.

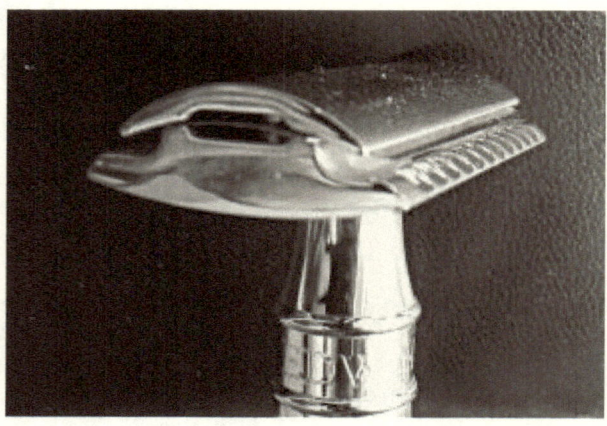

Close up of my razor head. See the part in the middle that looks kind of like an old fashioned phone? If you look close you can see the thin line of the razor. It rests between the top cap and the bottom safety bar (the scalloped looking thing running the length of the head). The top and bottom bar ensure that only a thin amount of the razor is exposed to skin, which you can see if you look close (the razor is a slightly different shade, flush with the top bar).

Shaving was cool for me right up until the time that I actually had to start doing it seriously, and then it got lame quick. It was time consuming, expensive, and generally annoying. When I found out about DE shaving though my interest was piqued for a simple reason, cost. While the startup cost would be more, the idea of not having to spend a ton of money on razor cartridges anymore was incredibly appealing. Buying my razor was justified to myself through reasoning that if it worked out I'd save a lot of money in the long run.

Since I've started though, cost has become a minor issue to me (though I still think it will be cheaper, which I'm quite happy about). Now, the two main reasons I'm doing it are that it gives me a much better shave, and it's a lot of fun. The better shave part is simple: my shaves are closer, with less irritation (not that I had much before, but noticeable on cold days), and the shave last longer. With cartridges, by the afternoon my face was getting scruffy and by dinner if I wanted to look nice when going out I almost needed to shave again. A good shave now will almost last me until the next morning.

And, as I said, it's just more fun. Why do people build computers rather than just buying one from the store, change their own oil, make workshops in their garage, or buy sewing machines? Because there's satisfaction and enjoyment to be had from doing a job yourself. Watching something go from start to finish, building skills and talents so that the next time is better than the last, seeing a result and feeling personally connected to the result because of the effort and attention you put into it. Those are feelings you can't buy, only earn, and they are worth having.

Shaving this way allows me to have those feelings every morning, and feel the results throughout the day. Shaving with a cartridge now just seems like bowling with the bumpers up.

So that's why I'm doing this. Is it cheaper? Yes, for me I think it will be. Is it a better shave? Yes, for me I know that it is. Is it enjoyable? Absolutely! It's turned a chore into an enjoyable ritual, what more could I ask for?

Picking My Razor: Three Piece Suits Me

January 23, 2014

I don't buy for myself easily. Law school credit for moot court participation should really be given to me anytime I spend more than about $5 on something I want. Wills have been given serious consideration and reached their final conclusion in less time than I've spent deciding if I want to buy a $1 app for my phone.

So despite the potential financial savings of switching to a DE razor, it still took me weeks to come to a conclusion. A substantial part of that was spent deciding which razor I wanted, which in turn was also trying to convince myself that spending money in the first place was actually worthwhile by finding the razor that justified it the most.

Complicating this was the fact that there are TONS of options. These razors have been around for over a century, and so there are hundreds of types floating about in the internet ether available for purchase. They range from models introduced this year, to vintage razors that predate my parents. Razors that are mainly plastic and cost a few dollars, to razors that, based on their cost, must have been carved out of unicorn horn in the forges of Mordor.

My first step was simple: I asked on Facebook. Turns out several friends were already shaving like this, and so their input and suggestions were an invaluable place to start.

I wanted something that I felt would last me a long time, many years hopefully. Changing to a whole new setup only to have the razor break would be extremely frustrating, or worse missing a great experience because I tried to cut corners on equipment, but so would spending a fortune only to find out that I couldn't stand DE shaving and wanted to go back to cartridge.

Using their tips I turned to amazon, and quickly settled on three brands: Parker, Merkur, and Edwin Jagger. All had excellent reviews, looked great, and were within the price range I'd set for myself ($40 or less). But between these three brands are dozens of models, so I had to dig a bit deeper.

The first to get ruled out were the Parkers, for two reasons. First, I decided that I wanted an all metal razor. Something that looked and felt like it was crafted out of the fender of a classic American land barge. The Parkers looked dang snazzy with the black faux ebony handles, but I wanted something a bit different.

The second reason deals with the mechanics. There are three types of DE razors: two piece, three piece, and butterfly. Two piece razors have half the head permanently mounted to the handle, with a rod running through the shaft from base to head. The rod screws into the top head piece, locking the two pieces together with the razor between them. Three piece razors have a handle, bottom head/ safety bar, and top head piece. Rather than a rod that screws from the base, the three piece screws in at the top edge of the handle. A butterfly razor has a permanently mounted head that opens like a Venus fly trap, the razor is deposited inside and then it closes back up on it.

I decided early on that I didn't want a butterfly styled razor. While they are reviewed well and have been around for decades, I wanted as few moving parts as possible. There are fewer things to break, less things to get gummed up with hair and soap, etc. Honestly I have no idea if that's even a significant issue with those razors. But the mental image was in my mind, so I decided just to avoid have the brain itch and just focus on to the other two.

After a good amount of asking and searching, it came down to the Merkur 34c and the Edwin Jagger de89L (the De89 Barely was my favorite, but I couldn't justify the extra expense simply for a different handle pattern). They both had a lot going for them. The Merkur 34c was recommended by a friend who loves his, and from everything I've read it is one of the benchmarks by which other razors are now compared. All metal, small, weighty, industrial styled and a two piece, it's the Willy Jeep of modern shaving.

The Edwin Jagger de89L is relatively new, having been out for only a few years. It uses the same three-piece head design as the more expensive Muhler razors, with a lined, grooved handle that has a more classic style. While not as widely reviewed as the Merkur, it seemed to compare well and the company had some excellent reviews concerning their customer service (sending hand written apology letter when errors were found, etc.). Plus, it was on sale at the time bringing it just under the Merkur in price.

I bounced between the two for probably a week and a half before committing, and I have not had a single regret. I love the feel of it in my hand, the weight of the metal, and the solid feel that it has when taking it apart or putting it back together. It feels like it was built to last.

What finally tipped the scales for me was that I liked the three piece design. While it has more pieces it has no moving parts, which I really liked. Though my friends assured me that they'd never had any issue with water or soap building up in the Merkur's hollow handle, in the back of my mind I knew it was going to bug me on top of all the other stresses of trying to figure out how to use it and take care of it properly.

That being said, I wouldn't mind picking one up down the line. Now that I'm getting a little more comfortable with things, and have a razor that I love, a little experimentation wouldn't be a bad thing. But given the cost, that'll probably have to wait a few years.

Till then I'll be enjoying my Jagger. Worth every penny!

What the Heck is a BBS, and Other Vexing Issues.

January 26, 2014

Friday was probably the worst shave I've had since I started this whole escapade. I don't know what happened, but my face got tore up. It was not good, but luckily for me all bleeding stopped with a cold water wash.

Really, shaving that whole week was pretty lousy. I'm using a new brand of blade from the mix, Astra. Was it that I was getting over confident? Was the blade too sharp or too dull for how I'd been shaving? Was it just a bad blade in the batch? I don't know, but all day Friday my face was tender and there were some noticeable red spots on my neck.

It served as an important reminder to me of something I've said all along: I have no idea what I'm doing. Right now I'm the guy who's read about how to water-ski without ever getting on a boat, and now is trying to get up for the first time.

A reminder of this also came while I was perusing some shave blogs, and I noticed everyone saying "BBS." I had no idea what that acronym meant, and while that's a normal feeling in DC where everything is acronymed I thought in this case I ought to figure out what they were talking about. Turns out BBS means "baby butt smooth," the pinnacle of shaving smoothness that can be obtained.

While I haven't ever gotten that all around, I've had it in a few spots and boy does it feel smooth. I guess that's a good goal to work towards. Today's shave, also using Astra blades, is excellent. Smooth, no bleeding, close, and my face feels great. Two passes, one with the grain, re-lather, and then one against. Took extra time and paid close attention to the blade angle, trying to get as little tug as possible. At times it felt like the razor wasn't even in contact but rather the safety bar was simply wiping away the hair and lather.

Excellent!

While I might end up spending more money as it becomes a hobby than I would when it was just a chore, it's nice to remind myself that it's a hobby grounded in a good financial basis. While cheaper cartridges could be probably found, especially if I went with off brand or Dollar Shave Club, it's nice to see that great shaves can be had for less than 10 cents a blade.

Grains, GRAINS!

January 28, 2014

While improvements have doubtlessly been made since I picked up DE shaving, I'm still working out what exactly I'm doing with all this. So far there's only one part of it all that I feel confident I've got locked down, and that's changing razor blades.

As I've mentioned before, a lot of shave blogs advise that you shave at least once with the grain before going against. I've been experimenting with this, and I'll admit that it does give a rather nice shave.

For day to day shaving though, I'm finding myself returning to my previous method: full lather, one slow and attentive pass against the grains, then a very quick with the grains pass (no lather, water or something on the face if anything) just to make sure I didn't miss anything and to try and keep it all even.

While I've never seen any websites advise such a technique, and while time may teach me why, it works for me. And that, I think, is the wonderful thing about DE shaving: you are much more personally involved in what you're doing. Every face is different, and while there are fundamentals to learn at the end of the day it's all about what works for you. As you're more closely involved in what you're doing, you naturally pick up on what works best.

In my case ingrown hairs and razor burn aren't a problem, so I can shave this way and it works great for me. I'll still be using the beard reduction method when I've not shaved for a day or two, or when there's something important and I really want a close and smooth shave, but for day to day I'll probably go with my traditional method.

On a related note: I'm still working out how to get a good lather. The two methods I've been using are lather on your hand and lather directly on your face, and both have been coming up a bit short lately. I think I'm not loading my brush as much as I have been, so that's something I'll need to work on.

Review: Astra Superior Platinum

January 31, 2014

Part of me wishes these had not worked even slightly well, then I could have used the joke "Astra-ick." With that joke out of the way, let's move on to how I almost cut my face off because I'm too cheap to throw away a used 9¢ blade that I didn't even like:

As part of the on going experiment, the last two weeks I've been using Astra Superior Platinum razor blades. Made in Russia, they are one of the brands that I knew about prior to starting DE shaving due to a former professor of mine recommending them. I was thus tempted to start using them as my first blade for the trial, but I wanted to get a bit more experience and comparison under my belt first so that I'd hopefully enjoy them more as well as have a more impartial experience.

Unlike Shark blades there are, of course, no sharks on the packaging. While certainly disappointing, this is completely understandable.

That being said, I went into it really wanting to like them, not the least reason of which is that you can buy a box of 100 of them for the cost of a movie ticket.

The first week, simply, did not go well. The shaves were bad, both in result and in the fact that they just weren't that enjoyable. Shaving wasn't smooth, nor did my face feel such afterward, and I noticed that my face felt much drier than usual. Within a couple hours of shaving things would be feeling sharp and bristly. It hit bottom around Friday when I had what was probably the worst shave in years, with a good amount of blood and discomfort. Had the cold rinse and aftershave not stopped it, I would have taken a picture. It was not good.

By the end of the week I was disliking them so much that I was ready to cut their trial period short and move on to something else. But, after thinking on it more I decided to go one more week for a couple reasons:

1. It was a weird week, and definitely not normal circumstances. There were snow days, snow delays, and general disruption of the morning schedule. Maybe that threw me off.
2. It might have just been a bad blade.
3. It's just one more week, and it'll give you more information.

So with some trepidation I set a new blade, steeled my nerves, and set out on a second week. Luckily and happily, it went a lot better. I made extra efforts to make sure I was lathering well, and that I wasn't rushing things. Most important, I paid closer attention to the angle of the blade than I have in weeks, trying to make sure that I wasn't being too aggressive. This extra attention paid off, and while the fun factor didn't go up much the shaves definitely improved. By the end of the trial I was consistently getting shaves I was satisfied with, but never thrilled.

So how do they stack up? They seemed to hold up fairly well, perhaps getting a bit dull toward the end of the week. But I found myself neither enjoying the shave nor enjoying the results as much as I did with the Shark blades. Shark seemed to give me a slightly closer, smoother, more even and longer lasting shave while also leaving my face feeling better.

Astra does stack up favorably against Derby in some regards, giving what felt to be a closer shave in most places. But Derby's shave simply felt better, and as a result I noticed that when I didn't shave everyday the growth seemed to be more even and comfortable than Astra provides.

Despite really wanting to like them, I just didn't have a great experience with Astra. I'm sure they are a fine blade for many people, but for me it just didn't work out...this time. I still have three blades, and later in the experiment I'll return to them and see if and how things have changed. Perhaps with more experience, or warmer summer months, things will be different.

Conclusion: I got mixed results, both good and bad. So, right now I'm going with good, with an Astra-ick.

Bam, that joke just came full circle.

True Grit – How DE Shaving Gets You a Better Scruff

February 3, 2014

Unexpected consequences sometimes result in important discoveries, like penicillin, chocolate chip cookies, or Miracle Whip.

My goal in switching to safety razors was to find a cheaper, better way to shave. In that regard: mission accomplished. There has emerged an interesting but wholly unexpected consequence though: a better gruff.

Now, I'm a man who is not unfamiliar with the ways of the facial hair. True fact: for about a year prior to my starting this Amanda used to be able to tell what day of the week it was by the amount of growth I was sporting. That's because unless I had work I would shave on Sundays for church and then just let it go during the week. While I'm not the hairiest guy around, I've got a respectable amount and it comes in fairly quick.

Most guys have heard the stories that shaving makes your hair grow in thicker and darker. I don't buy that, not because of any actual biological proof but because it just doesn't make any kind of sense to me. But, DE shaving has given me an appreciation at least for why some people might think that because shaving properly does do one important thing: it makes your hair feel like it's growing in better.

I don't know why it is, but here's my theory: the closer, better shave results in hair that's more evenly and more cleanly cut than from cartridges. Rather than sharply cut, uneven hair that grows in like gravel landscaping, a good DE shave results in scruff that grows in like a good medium grit sand paper. Rough but with an even smoothness quality. That's a man's shadow.

Anyone who's ever tried to grow grass knows that a good lawn starts with good preparation (or sod), and that good maintenance means that it'll keep growing healthy. The better you cut the grass, the better it'll look for days afterward as it starts growing back. Do yourself a favor and give your face the same attention. I'm not saying it's as good as penicillin, but you'll hopefully be using it on a more regular basis.

Foam Slinging: How to Lather Like Someone who Doesn't Know What They're Doing.

February 5, 2014

Occasionally my school does an externship fair, where all sorts of law offices come in seeking externs (like an intern, but less coffee fetching). Hundreds of students print up their resumes, dress up in their most lawyerly looking clothes, and go out there to try and win themselves some work. While wandering through the hallway during one I saw an interesting situation: a student had apparently either tied his tie wrong, or had it come undone and he didn't know how to re-tie it, so one kindhearted faculty member was hurriedly trying to fix it for him.

I could empathize, while I learned a while ago how to tie one properly (having had to ask for help myself more than a few times) I'm currently going through a similar experience: finding out that I don't know much about shaving cream. For a brief moment where I thought I'd figured out how to properly lather. I was creating a good amount of rich foam, it spread well, and protected great. That lasted two or three days, and then for the two weeks following I found myself getting a lesson in humility.

I think a lot of it had to do with that I still haven't worked out a process that works well for me, and that I don't know much about the steps involved. So, I went back to school (so to speak) and turned to the internet for help. The last few days have shown a marked improvement, and while I think I have a long way to go I do think I'm on the right path now. So, without further ado, here is the method I've worked out for lathering (using shave soap):

1. I start by soaking my brush in warm water for a couple minutes, placing it bristle down in a mug and filling to about the handle. I also drip some water onto the top of the shave soap bar, just enough to get it wet, to help warm and soften it.
2. After soaking I shake out my brush, trying to leave enough water in the bristles for it to be wet but not much that it is dripping of soaked. Basically, getting the water out that's easy to get out. Two or three shakes.
3. I then "load" the brush with soap. I was previously doing this by wiping the brush on the shave soap like a paint brush, but I am now doing moderate pressure circular motions, primarily in the middle of the bristles but occasionally rotating the brush to get the edges. If it starts getting bubbles on the soap block then I try to remove a bit of the water, rather I try to get a thicker goo.
4. I don't have a lather bowl, so I first apply directly to the face. Usually a pretty light coat if I'm doing a two pass shave, as the first pass will be with the grain and that doesn't need a whole lot of foam to keep the skin happy.
5. For the second lather I use my hand to mix up a thicker foam, using circular motions and

occasionally squeezing out the brush between my thumb and for finger. This pulls thick lather from the middle, which is then applied to the face with the brush. While the lather directly on the face method feels good for it's light abrasiveness, applying already lathered foam makes for a soft and slick conclusion.

Is this how you're supposed to do it? Darned if I know, but it works for me. You can spend a year researching every possible method, but at the end of the day you've just got to dive in and start trying stuff out. Besides, it's not like it's anything that can't be undone with the run of a tap.

Shaving on the Fly: Helpful Tips to Avoid Looking Like You Hitchhiked.

February 10, 2014

A good double edge (DE) razor is a fine tool, and I have no desire to go back to cartridge razors. But I believe in giving credit where credit is due, and so I'll note one notable advantage cartridge razors have over DE: I've never had a problem taking them in a carry-on bag on an airplane. Since a DE blade by design can easily be removed from the razor, for the time being they can only be brought on a plane in checked baggage. That's no problem if you're bringing a suitcase along, but if you're like me then you prefer to travel with just a backpack or small carry on bag. Assuming you intend on obeying the rules, that means you've either got to skip shaving for the trip duration or find an alternative solution. For Christmas we went back west to visit family, so I ran into that very problem. I figured that I had a few options, among them:

- I could bring my old Mach 3. It would work just fine, but I kinda liked DE shaving so I wanted to avoid that option if possible.
- There are internet forums to connect volunteers that help out fellow DE shavers who are traveling by meeting up with them somewhere and giving them a blade to use during their trip. This seemed strange, weird,

and a bit creepy to me, so while I applaud the generosity of those who do it I didn't feel like doing so myself.

- Of course, there are drug stores all over the place so I could just but a blade once I got there. This would mean though that I would have a bunch left over that couldn't be brought back on the plane, thus being costly and wasteful.

Finally I settled on a simple solution: I'd just mail myself one. While this wouldn't have worked if I was staying in a hotel (unless they accepted mail for upcoming guests), staying with family allowed me to do some advance work. I just took an old plastic razor package, taped the end so the blade wouldn't slide out, *(add and)* then dropped it in a letter with a stamp about a week before I left. Just be sure if you do this that you mail the blade safely. Razors ship by mail all the time so it's not inherently unsafe, but you don't want the razor cutting its way through the envelope or injuring a postal worker. That's why I used the plastic package that the razor had shipped in, kept the blade from getting lost, broken, or hurting anyone.

Just think about it, planes full of guys that have neither beards nor shaves, just gnarly haired growth. *shudder*

It worked out great. Before I left I took the blade out of my razor, making it both safe and acceptable to fly with, and by the time I landed in SLC there was a new blade waiting for me. Once the trip was over I just threw the blade away and flew back. Everyone was happy, I got a great shave while on the road, and no one had to worry that Mountain Man McGee was sitting next to them on the airplane.

Uh-Oh: First Blood

February 11, 2014

It's been a good run, but after three months I finally found myself with my first bleeder. While I've seen spots of blood before, I decided that I wouldn't count anything that stopped with or before a cold water wash and aftershave. Today's nick survived two cold water washes and aftershave, so while it actually isn't too bad it technically makes the cut (har-har):

It should be of no surprise that this occurred on the morning of my first interview for post-graduate work, because when else would be better? Luckily it's not actually that bad, and by the time breakfast was over it had closed up. A wipe with water and you can't even tell it was there. No where near as bad as the one and only time I cut myself with a Mach3, which left three parallel lines along my cheek for the next few days.

But, rest assured this will be noted in the razor blade review. I'm sure that the company will be disappointed to know this, as they were doing really well so far, and an obscure book will likely have significant impact on their Q1 earnings.

Review: Personna Platinum Chrome (Red IP)

February 14, 2014

Made of Swedish steel and manufactured in Israeli, perhaps it's fitting that during the Olympics I'd get to try out the Personna Platinum Chrome blades (in my British razor, no less!).

First things first, these things take an effort to track down. For the sake of this review (and the book) I'll just call them Personnas or Personna Reds, but you've got to be careful when looking around online. Personna is the brand, and they seem to be related to the brand Crystal, I think it's sort of a Chevy/ GMC thing. And different Personna blades are sold under very similar names, depending on what country they are made and/ or sold in.

Just plopping the name into Amazon turns up these blades. Those are not the same ones that I've been using. I've been I've been using the Platinum Red Pack found on Bullgooseshaving.com.

And boy, these things are sharp. Even with a couple days growth they cut clean with minimal effort. About the only time I noticed any pulling or catching was around the front edge of my chin, and that was quickly resolved with a touch of extra shaving cream. Otherwise it cut nice and smooth, especially with the mustache and side-burn areas.

Not only are they sharp, they are fun to shave with. After the rough two weeks that the Astra blades gave me I was feeling a bit burned out on shaving, but these guys got me back in the spirit. I found myself quickly looking forward to shaving again, though I did find myself wanting to get an extra day's growth every so often just so I'd have more to do in the morning.

There was however a downside. It felt like the Personna blades seemed to either dull more quickly than other blades, or that they didn't quite perform as well with daily shaving as what other blades have. While a two day scruff seemed to shave off smooth and easily, a day to day shave seemed to have spots that were a little rough or scratchy. And they did give me my first significant bleeder, though that might have just been my nerves since it was a big day. I don't know if this was a result of bad blades, poor technique, observer bias, or just how they are, but I'll be looking closely at it when I revisit them later.

Price wise they are a bit more expensive than the other blades I've been using. But the difference when spread out over the weeks amounts to a difference of dimes, so nothing that's going to be breaking the bank. While they can be difficult to track down they can be bought in bulk from Bullgoose, who I'm already a fan of, so availability and supply shouldn't be an issue.

So how do they stack up? Right now they are sitting second in my personal ranking, just behind Shark

Super Stainless. I liked substantially more than Astra, and while I enjoyed Derby quite a bit and perhaps felt a touch better, the Personna shaved closer and more even. But Sharks still seem to have given me a shave that was as close or closer, and my face just felt fresher and smoother afterward.

I've still got eight Personna blades though so I'll definitely be revisiting them later in the year. I look forward to comparing them more directly with Shark and any other rising challengers. I haven't worked out exactly how that'll be done, but I suspect that Personna will be a strong competitor.

While there was a couple of issues, (no comma) these blades are slick, sharp, and smooth.

Finding Shaving Stuff

February 21, 2014

It seems ironic to me that were it not for the internet, a late 20th century invention that exploded in the 21st, I would not be shaving with something designed in the 19th. English majors or Alanis Morrissette may disagree with whether I used the term right, but my point remains: even though this was probably common when my dad was growing up I'd never heard of it until my late 20's. While I knew about straight razor shaving, I figured everything there was about shaving was what was found in a typical grocery store aisle. My, how wrong I was.

While I don't fault stores for not stocking more double-edge (DE) razors, blades, or various shaving products beyond barbersol and gels, they are in it to make a profit after all, it does help create a false belief that there isn't anything else out there. Razor manufacturers seem happy to perpetuate perception, presumably because cartridge razors have higher profits. Case in point: Gillette manufactures a dozen types of DE razor blades, including the one that I am using now (Gillete 7 O'Clock Sharpedge). Wilkinson Sword/ Schick, Gillette's major competitor, makes a dozen of their own.

Go on their websites and try to find any mention of it. As far as I can tell they not only will not sell them in their online store, they won't even suggest they exist.

But that's not to say there aren't great places to find products. Here are a few places I've found that carry traditional shaving products:

- The Art of Shaving- Owned by P&G, who also own Gillette, you can find these at malls or other upper scale shopping areas. When I was first getting into DE shaving they helped show me how to properly hold the razor. I've never seen them carry more than a couple kinds of DE blades (Merkur and Gillette), and only a few handles. Prices are a touch high, but it's a brick and mortar store so it makes up for it with having actual people there to work with you.
- Drug stores- I've seen DE razor blades at about half of the CVS stores I've looked in, but it is usually just one or two kinds. Every CVS I've looked in carries a handful of older shaving products (aftershave, cream, shaving soap, basic brush). I would imagine Walgreens has similar stock. Keep your eyes open for smaller, older, independent stores that are trying to sell hit the market and products that the corporate stores are overlooking.
- Tobacconists- I don't know about cigarette stores, but if you can find an old fashioned tobacco store (pipe, cigar) they tend to also carry some traditional shaving equipment. I guess it goes with the dapper image.
- Online- Of course, you can find anything online. Amazon, as always. Bullgoose Shaving has excellent prices and selection, and I've heard good things about Mama Bears

Soaps (which I'll probably be ordering from once my current soap runs low).
- Farmers Markets/ Renaissance Fair- Keep your eyes open for local markets where small producers of soaps or creams would be selling their products. I have not personally looked at the Ren Fair yet, but I know of one person who stocks up on shave soap when they come to town then uses it all year.
- Barber/ Shave Supply- Somewhat rare, they can still be found around.

Once you know where to look it doesn't take a lot of effort, the trick is finding the places with good prices and selection.

Cold Water, Cold Steel, and Your Face...Well, My Face.

February 26, 2014

In the classic war film "Dirty Dozen" the film's name is coined in a key scene: as the motley convicts are being trained they are forced to shave in cold water. Fed up with the unequal treatment between them and the guards they refuse to shave until hot water is provided, banding together as a team for the first time. Rather than giving in to their demands they are instead told by their commanding officer that they'll be spending the time normally used for shaving doing more training. As they aren't going to be clean shaven, they are thus called the dirty dozen.

I never understood why cold water was an issue to them. While I didn't use it myself I didn't use particularly warm water either. Virtually every shaving guide I've seen says that hot water should be used, and so that's what I've primarily used since adopting double-edge (DE) shaving. But on rare occasions I've seen suggestions that cold water could be equally effective.

Though we live in a world where hot water availability is the norm, there are plenty of reasons a cold shave might be the only option. (Though we live in a world where hot water availability is the norm, there are plenty of reasons a cold shave might be the only option.) Perhaps the water heater is broken, there was a power outage, you're out camping, zombie apocalypse, or the tank isn't big enough to provide hot water for everyone who needs to get cleaned up. There's all sorts of reasons that being used to cold shaving would be beneficial.

So I decided to give it a try, and for the last few days I've been used cold water before, during, and after my shave. The results have been very encouraging.

The shave itself does not seem to be suffering substantially. While I do think it is slightly rougher, the difference is very small. For day to day shaving purposes, where I'm just trying to get cleaned up and out the door, it is perfectly acceptable. In fact, there seems to be less irritation and slight bleeding from where the blade has cut a bit too close. That seems to be the trade off: slightly less smooth, but slightly easier on the skin.

I have noticed one problem with cold water shaving though: lather and hair gets stuck easier in the blade and razor. I think this is due to the temperature thickening the lather, and even running it under the tap meant that much of it wouldn't come out easily. So, I came up with a cheater solution: I would use hot water to rinse off the blade, breaking down the lather that had built on it, then cool it back off with cold water before shaving again. While that might not be a pure cold water shave, it made it loads easier.

Finally, the cold water seemed to give a better lather. Perhaps, as above, that's because the cooler lather was naturally thicker, but for whatever reason it seemed to apply thicker and last longer. I'm going to be very tempted to keep up the cooler lather, if nothing else.

Refreshing wise it was different experience than warm, but not necessarily bad. I think of the two warm water was slightly more enjoyable, but cold definitely gave a good invigorating feeling. I think it probably boils down to whether you're the type to splash warm or cold water on your face, or what type of mood you're in. While I normally loathe cold water, I found it a brisk and enjoyable change of pace.

Will I switch over completely? Probably not, but I'm not going to rule out doing it either. Rather, like different razors, soaps, aftershaves, and creams, I think it's going to be a valuable option in deciding what shave I'm in the mood for that day. I've found it to give a great, enjoyable, and refreshing shave. What more can you ask for?

Review: Gillette 7 O'clock Sharpedge

March 1, 2014

For as cool a name as "Sharpedge" is, it does seem rather redundant. It's a razor blade after all, a double edged one at that. You'd think it would have a sharp edge by nature, preferably two. But still, I like the name. What does the 7 O'clock have to do with anything? Heck if I know. There seems to be a whole line of them, so it must be working for them.

But the name doesn't lie, these things can cut, which brings us to our latest review! For the last two weeks I've been using the Sharpedges to see how they shave, as part of the on going experiment. Made in St. Petersberg Russia I found these blades to be sharp, slick, and a pleasure to use.

When proper time and attention was given to get a good two pass shave, I found these blades gave a close, smooth, great feeling result. In fact, while I don't know whether it was the blades or just improving skills but I think that off all the blades I've tried thus far I had the least amount of spot bleeding or irritation with the Sharpedges.

There was a couple of drawbacks. First, they didn't seem to give very good one pass, against the grain shaves. Granted, not many do, but I seemed to notice it more with the Sharpedges. I don't know if that's because it actually doesn't shave as well, or if I notice it more because it shaves so well with two passes (one with the grain then one against) that I just happen to notice the difference more. Regardless, notice it I did, and while it wasn't a bad shave at all it was one that by mid-afternoon things were getting scratchy.

Second, there seemed to be some inconsistency sharpness and how well the blades held an edge. I tried to shave pretty evenly, with each side getting roughly the same use, but with each blade there always seemed to be one side that simply shaved better and one that was a bit more struggle, even if it had been used less. When things would start pulling with that side using the other always solved the problem. It seemed to happen with both blades, so when I use the rest of them later I'll be keeping my eye on them.

How did they rank up? I think they might be challenging the Shark Super Stainless for my favorite blade. I'll need to do a closer comparison between the two (and any others that are competing for the top spot), but I found them extremely comfortable, effective, and user friendly. Even when I started getting a bit sloppy they seemed to treat my skin well, and that's a result that's hard to argue with. I think I enjoyed the Sharks a bit more, but they were also very early so I'll need to test them later and see how much of that was the razor and how much was the user.

Verdict: An excellent blade, one of my favorites thus far. I'd rate it above the Personna, Astra, and Derby, possibly in the top position that Shark Stainless has been holding.

I approve.

<u>Old Fashioned Shaving in a Sarcastic World</u>

March 5, 2014

Monday morning I did something that I would have never imagined doing prior to five months ago: I shaved on a snow day.

I mean, who does that? Granted, prior to a few years ago I wouldn't have imagined having a snow day in the first place, but that's small potatoes compared to the larger point: I made the effort to shave when I was neither going out nor even just entertaining guests. For me, that's weird.

Or it was weird, I should say. Things have changed, both my attitude toward the matter and the way in which I do it. After a life time of shaving with multi-bladed cartridges, I switched to an old fashioned, single blade, double-edge razor. What prompted the change was simple: double-edge razor blades cost as little as 6-7 cents each. That's right, *cents*. I figured at that price I'd be crazy not to give it a try.

But that's not why I stuck with it. Double-edge shaving takes effort. It takes skill. It takes practice, practice, practice. And even when you're good at it, a bit of casualness or carelessness and you're risking a real bleeder, a rough face, or both.

When I was contemplating buying my first double-edge razor I didn't know that, though I did realize it was going to take more work and attention. I did have one thought on my mind:

"I hope this doesn't make me a hipster..."

Now, if you're of the hipster variety then that's your business. But, I didn't want to go down that road, where things are done for sarcasm's sake. I didn't want my morning to start off with ironic pleasure at the fact that I'm shaving in 2014 with something invented over a hundred years ago. I wanted to shave my face, not indulge in uniqueness just so I could be different. That's not me, nor do I want it to be (existentially, perhaps this was just double downing on things by doing something that some might see as ironic, but then finding a reason to do it other than the sarcastic reason they expect, but since I just thought of that five months in I don't know that I'm that clever).

It worried me, not enough so that I didn't do it but enough so that I wondered what was really in it for me. Sure, it saves money, but was that all there was to it? Maybe at first, but since I've started I've found a much more important reason: satisfaction.

Satisfaction can come in a lot of ways. It can mean that something has meet the basic requirement, and thus the result, while perhaps not great, is satisfactory. It can mean that you'll soon be dueling a Southern gentleman. For me, in this context, I think I can best describe it as some combination of pleasure and fulfillment. There might be a better word for that feeling out there, but I'll settle for this one until I find it.

I'm not saying that old fashioned shaving has fulfilled all my hopes and dreams, filled a missing spot in my life, or changed my outlook on world poverty. It's shaving for crying out loud. But is helping me develop appreciation for something that as I get older I'm finding more and more applicable in many parts of my life: the value of doing things in a slower, more patient, more attentive manner. The value of effort when effort isn't needed.

I was never a gearhead, never got into wood or metal working, and if I had perhaps I'd have come to this conclusion sooner. Perhaps I just needed to age enough to appreciate it. But much like someone wants to change their own oil, or adjust timing, build themselves a bookshelf, or what have you, I've found that there is both enjoyment and satisfaction to be had in taking the personal approach. Knowing your tools, evaluating your need, focusing on the work, and then reaping the rewards of a job well done.

Sure, you might get a good job done faster and easier if you spent a bit more money. To some that would be money well spent, just as I spend more on certain things I don't particularly enjoy doing rather than doing them myself. But the time and effort is paying off in forming what has become a relaxing morning ritual, a way to transition to the focus and professional mindset that the day requires.

And that's where the sarcasm has no place. While I'm sure there are plenty of people out there shaving with a double-edge, single edge, or straight razor who are doing it as some ironic expression or sarcastic stunt so they can feel different or better than someone else, for me it is much simpler. It's fun, it's cheap (unless the hobby factor takes over), it's a great shave, and it takes effort.

In my rush to save time, to get more done faster, to be more efficient, I lose sight too often of the value that steady, patient effort can have on the soul. But I'm getting it back, one morning at a time.

Review: Col. Conk's Shave Soap – Bayrum

March 10, 2014

While there's plenty of shave sites out there that will bemoan the inferior nature of aerosol shaving cream, I've never had a problem with it. It's fast, it's simple, it's consistent, it's never given me any problems, and when the time came to make the switch to double-edge shaving I picked up a travel size can. It did the job, but after weeks of researching razors I'd gotten a hankering to try out making my own lather. So for Christmas my wife got me a badger hair brush and a puck of Col. Conk's Glycerin Shave Soap, and off I went.

I've been using Col. Conk's for two months now, and I've been greatly enjoying it. It took several weeks to really get the hang of what I was doing, and then several more weeks to get the method refined to the point that I'm getting consistent lathers. But I've greatly enjoyed the soap, and while I might get a can of aerosol or shave gel to have around in case I'm running late, I have no desire to go back to regular use of either of them.

The soap has a rich, solid smell to it. I'd never heard of bay rum before, but I'm now a fan. The soap, and by extension the lather, smells like something you'd find in an old, wood paneled barbershop. Thick, rich, smooth. While the scent seems like it's diminished over the last month or so, that may be because I've gotten so used to it that I just don't notice it as much. I shave in a smaller guest bathroom, and the soap has given the room a wonderful smell just by being in there. While I would like to try some of the menthol or sandlewood soaps out there, I'm going to have a hard time not buying another bay rum product.

The soap has also held up to daily use very well. I'm about two and a half months into using it everyday, and I suspect that I can easily get another several weeks out of it. The only problem I anticipate with getting easily another month is that I might wear through the middle of the puck, but if I load the brush from the edges then I should be fine. More experience will tell me whether this is a sizable amount of time for soap to last, or if either the soap or my loading method are reducing it faster than normal, but I have no complaints with how it's held up.

The soap produces a good lather that makes for a great shaving experience. My method of loading from it has been this: I soak my brush for a minute or two in warm water, with a few drops of water dripped on the top of the soap puck to help soften things. After shaking out the water I do counter-clockwise circles until a brush has a good, somewhat thick paste of soap on it, then with a touch of water on the brush I lather directly on the face. Normally, a loading makes enough that I can make two applications for two shave passes.

The first application tends to be a bit thin. The lather tends to be pretty low, and looks more thick soapy than shaving cream. After the first pass with the razor I add a touch more water to the brush and start reapplying, this time squeezing the brush through my thumb and forefinger to pull out some soap lather. I lather up the brush tips on what's been squeezed out, and then apply to face. This time it's thick, solid foam that really hangs on. Since this is normally my against the grain pass, this thicker lather is really helpful both to protect the skin and to help me see where I've shaved and where I haven't, as at this point the hair is getting short enough to make it hard to tell in spots. At the end of the shave, it left the face feeling smooth, clean, and soft.

Frankly, while I want to try new products there's a part of my that is perfectly satisfied with what I've found and wouldn't mind sticking with it. This is a solid soap that I am happy to recommend. It smells great, it lasts a long time, and it does an excellent job where it counts the most: on the face. While I don't know that it helped give me a closer shave than aerosol creams or gels, it absolutely gave me a better shave experience.

I am sold.

Review: Shark Super Chrome

March 14, 2014

Just to lay it out there at the outset: I have no idea what the difference is between the Shark Super Stainless razor blades I tried a couple months ago and the Shark Super Chrome that I tried this week.

That's not hyperbole, I honestly don't. I've looked around online, and there doesn't seem to be any real consensus. About half the people out there think there's no difference at all, and about half think that the Super Stainless are a touch Sharper while the Chrome are a touch smoother.

The blades themselves look absolutely identical, and both say "Shark Super Stainless" on them. As far as I can tell the only difference is that the Stainless come in a paper box, and have two simple paper wrappers on them, while the Chrome comes in a plastic box, and has one nicely printed wrapper on it.

Interestingly, the price is not the same: Super Stainless currently cost $10.95 for 100, while Super Chrome cost $11.95 per 100. When not on sale, the Chrome only cost 4 cents more.

While they seem to be virtually identical, I find myself leaning toward the group that thinks there's a slight difference between the two. Shaving the last two weeks has been incredibly smooth. Not in the result on my face (though that wasn't bad), I feel like other razors like the 7 O'clock, Personna, and the

Super Stainless were better in that regard, but rather the Chrome seems to be incredibly forgiving, allowing for very forgiving shaving that just goes smoothly.

The blades being forgiving turned out to be an especially good thing as the blades seemed to lose their sharpness pretty quick. The first several shaves were excellent, but by the end of the week the shave quality seemed to drop noticeably. The result as my taking an increasingly aggressive approach with the blade, and while that is normally a recipe for disaster I hardly got so much as a spot of bleeding.

Which raises the question again: are these the same blades? I remember the Super Stainless being an excellent razor blade, and I don't recall a noticeable dip in quality. This leads to several theories:

1) They are the same blade, just packaged and marketed differently, and whatever differences I'm noticing are because my experience and expectations have changed.

2) They are the same blade, and any differences are simply a result of production variations.

3) They actually are different, and I'm noticing it.

This up coming week I'll be shaving with a Super Stainless blade so I can compare the two more directly, and will report back next week. While it's a deviation from the normal experiment timeline of two weeks a brand, I think that it'll be worth it for the sake of clarifying any differences between the two.

As for the Chrome itself, I enjoyed shaving with it. Is it the sharpest I've tried? Doesn't feel like it. But it does a solid job, gives a good shave, and is a breeze to use. A very good blade, but one that raises some questions that'll need more examination to answer.

Nerves of Steel

March 20, 2014

The first time I handled a double-edge safety razor blade you'd think I was trying to pick up a porcupine soaked in nitroglycerin. I'm like that with a lot of delicate things, or at least with things I think are delicate. The first time I built a computer I was convinced if I touched anything on the circuit board it would surely meltdown, or if I applied the slightest amount of pressure more than needed something would snap and my money would be gone. It's as though my brain thinks that any part of my finger other than the slightest edge of the fingertip is just waiting to shatter, snap, or incinerate anything it touches.

Now obviously I didn't think that I was going to destroy the razor blade by touching it wrong. That's silly. I apparently thought the slightest mishandling would result in a slice to the bone and massive blood loss. Gingerly I would unwrap the blades, and carefully load them into the razor with the skill, focus, and delicate determination of a bomb technician. It was a JOB.

As time and exposure has passed I now find myself much more comfortable. I still am wary of them, and that's probably good. When you stop respecting something that's when it's most likely to hurt you. But it's becoming increasingly normal, part of my regular shaving routine. Normality is funny like that.

The other night a fellow student mentioned he'd read my blog, and said that he was nervous to try it because he was worried about having a blade so exposed near his face. Now, I make plenty of jokes about how one day I'm going to cut my face off or cause some other serious harm, and it comes from a genuine understanding that there is a greater risk of injury shaving like this than with some alternative methods.

But at the same time it made me realize how far I've moved. My first time shaving with a safety razor I was nervous, and my hands might even have been shaking just a bit (an uncomfortable situation when you're trying not to cut yourself). Now, while I remain cautious and careful, the normality is increasingly setting in. My old fears increasingly seem silly or overwrought. Perhaps now, if I'm moving beyond my initial jitters, is the time when I can really start building skills. When I'm starting to know enough to have an idea about what I'm doing, but before long term habits have set in.

So if you're thinking about trying out traditional shaving, do it. Will you cut yourself? Maybe. Will it be serious? Probably not. You'll quickly realize that if a hundred million other people did it, you can too.

And it's a lot of fun. There's always that.

Comparison: Shark Super Stainless v. Shark Super Chrome

March 21, 2014

As I said last week, any differences that exist between Shark Super Stainless and Shark Super Chrome are not apparent from the outside. While they come in slightly different packaging, the razors themselves appear identical. This week I went back to Super Stainless to compare them when they're both fresh on my mind.

Aside from obvious differences in photo effort, from the outside there isn't much visual difference aside from one being packaged in plastic and the other not. However, after using the Stainless this week I feel confident in saying that there is a difference in the shave the two blades give.

The Chrome blade, as I said last week, is extremely easy to shave with. You almost have to try and cut yourself with it, it's that forgiving. Afterward, my skin always felt great, and on the first few shaves it kept things nice and close. However, it never got quite as close and smooth as what the other blades seemed to be able to give, and by the end of the week the blade was noticeably struggling.

The Stainless feels sharper, and throughout the week it gives a closer shave. By the end of the week, when the Chrome would be struggling, the Stainless both shaves closer and with less effort. However, it is a bit tougher on the skin, and while I never noticed any blood with a Chrome, with the Stainless it was not uncommon to see spots where a little blood had appeared. It always washed off with cold water though, never to return.

Personally, I like the Stainless much more. While the Chrome is a perfectly fine blade, I like the Stainless' sharpness and quality of shave. For a new shaver, I would recommend trying the Chrome first and then moving on to Stainless, while the later is in my opinion better I think the former would be a great blade for someone who is just building their skills and confidence.

First Impressions: That's Brisk Baby

March 23, 2014

After learning to lather with Col. Conks, I tried a different shaving soap for the first time today: Proraso Eucalyptus and Menthol. It came highly recommended from both friends and the internet, both for its quality and for the handy bowl that it comes in. After some warm water to open up the pores, I loaded the brush and went to work.

As the title implies, wow.

The lather goes on much smoother and silkier than I'm used to, I think this is because Proraso is a softer soap than the hard puck that I've gotten used to. After being used to bayrum scent of my previous soap this had a much sharper small to it. Not bad, but definitely different, like the smell of barbershop disinfectant.

Quickly I noticed something else I hadn't experienced before: it tingles. By the time I was fully lathered there was a distinct tingly feeling on my face, and as I shaved the spots where the lather was removed felt like a cool breeze on wet skin. It was very refreshing, and by the time I finished the second lather and pass my face was feeling almost a bit numb and puffy. A cold water rinse and some spice aftershave and I was feeling great. Even now, almost an hour later, I can still feel residual tingles.

The soap was accompanied with a brand new Treet brand razor blade. I've never used Treet before, but the razor did a great job delivering a close, smooth, even shave on two day old stubble. I can honestly say that this is the best feeling shave I've had in weeks, everything worked together for a great result. I'm really looking forward to more of this!

Money Down the Drain

March 28, 2014

While walking through CVS the other day I paused in the shaving aisle to see what I've been missing since switching to a double-edge safety razor. It seems that in my absence the situation has become even more bleak and frustrating.

I was shocked, for example, to see an eight pack of Fusion Proglide cartridges selling for nearly $40. That's over $4 each! That's crazy pants. Even the more sedate Mach3 cartridges were retailing for about $3 each, which while at one time I might have thought that to be reasonable now it just seems silly.

In contrast, there are Derby blades where you can get 200, yes, <u>two hundred</u> blades for fifteen bucks. 7.5 cents each, and enough to last you two years even if you were using two blades a week (I used one and got by just fine).

Granted, Derby isn't my favorite brand. But I liked them well enough, they shaved just as well as my Mach3 did and the price is a heck of a lot better.

I fault no one for using cartridges. If that's what you like and it works for your situation, then by all means, enjoy it. But personally, I'm glad to have found a new ship to sail on.

Sunday: The Best Shave of the Week

March 30, 2014

As my attitude toward shaving has slowly evolved from antipathy to anticipation, weekday shaving has increasingly become an enjoyable and satisfying experience. But, there remains one day a week which I always find myself most eager and excited to shave: Sunday. No other day compares to it, the shave always just feels better than usual, even when it probably actually isn't.

There may be a host of reasons for this, but I've narrowed it down what I think are the primary causes:

1) New razor blade- I've gotten in the habit of changing my razor blade on Saturday, after a week of shaving. Thus far that means one of two things, either Sunday is a brand new brand I've never experienced, or it means that I'm getting a fresh crack at my face using the experience I've built up with a brand throughout the week. Since DE razor blades each have their own strengths and qualities, one brand might shave quite different from another. Sunday means I get to build on what I've been learning, and apply it with a new, fresh blade.

2) More time- During the week I usually make breakfast for the wife and myself, while we're both rushing to get ready and out the door to work and

school. We budget our time well enough that it's rarely a mad rush, but it does mean that when I'm shaving in the morning there's a time frame that I've got to work in. Not on Sundays. On Sunday, I can take as much time as I like. It's quite, peaceful, and I can simply enjoy the experience. As Sunday is a day of religious observance to me, that peace is a welcome way to start the day.

3) Stubble- Like everyone else I know, my hair grows everyday. But since I shave most to everyday during the week, my daily shave tends to be about keeping things in check, maintenance. My shaves are much closer since switching to safety razors, and so while I've got some solid scruff by the next day (and occasionally the night before) it doesn't have a lot of time for growth between shaves. But, with my blade dull from a week of use, Saturday has become my day off from shaving. By the time Sunday rolls around I've got a couple days growth and, since stubble feels much coarser with safety razor shaves, I am looking forward to getting it cleaned up. More work to do, more satisfaction in the result.

Sunday isn't always the smoothest, it isn't always the closest or most even. I've had a few that were frankly just bad. But it's a rare day that Sunday isn't the most enjoyable shave of my week.

The Importance of Shaving During a Zombie Apocalypse

April 1, 2014

We've all been there: police stations overrun, hospitals a death trap, federal forces pulling back to mountain holdouts, bridges bombed, warlords rising, violence rampant, basically anytown America looking more and more like Chicago.

It's understandable to assume that now is not the time to worry about shaving. But you'd be wrong my friend...dead wrong. Here's why:

1) People with beards never fare well in apocalypse. Can't think of an example? That's cause there are none. Even heavy scruff is an indicator that things are going down hill. The Walking Dead folk, for example, are always scruffy, and what do they have to show for it? Misery, squalor, and desperation. Meanwhile, a clean shaven Charlton Heston in Omega Man and a clean shaven Will Smith in I Am Legend are living it up in penthouses, cruising in fancy cars, listening to their favorite music, plenty to eat, and living the good life.

2) A beard is bad for close combat. While Special Forces in Afghanistan have popularized the warrior beard, when it comes to hand to hand battles you want a clean maw. The reason? Because the last thing you want is for a zombie to grab a handful of beard hair. The Romans knew that (the grabbing

part, zombies debatable), and it was standard that Roman soldiers would go into battle shaved so as not to give the enemy something to grab onto.

3) It's aerodynamic. Whether you're running from shamblers or sprinters, cutting down on wind resistance can mean the difference between life and death.

4) Zombies don't shave. Well of course they don't, you say, so what? Well when you're approaching the barricades on the outskirts of a fortified encampment, that little bit of humanity might be just what you need to convince the sharpshooters your not a zed, and to hold their fire.

5) It's the secret to agrarian success. With industrial society collapsing we're headed back to the farm age. The pinnacle of that was reached in our country in the late 1700's. What did George Washington, Patrick Henry, Benjamin Franklin, Thomas Jefferson, John Adams, and the rest of our founding fathers have in common? Nary a beard on them, that's what.

So when you're scavenging your next burnt out storefront, snag yourself some razor blades. Civilization might be ending, but you've got a lot of living to do.

Creams and Soap: Getting a Good Morning Lather

April 3, 2014

When I first started using a safety razor I wasn't sold on also changing up my shaving cream. While I didn't normally use it, when I did I was perfectly happy with aerosol or gels, and it's what I used for the first month or so after switching razors. My wife thankfully had more foresight than I and got me a brush and shave soap for Christmas, I've been a believer ever since. It's opened up a whole new aspect to shaving, with hundreds of options available.

Most of those options fall into two groups: shaving creams, and shaving soaps.

So what's the difference? It's pretty simple:

Creams

Brush mixed shaving creams come in a tub or tube (like toothpaste), are fairly moist, and have the consistency of moderate to thick putty. My experience with creams has been that they are very easy to mix, and with a wet brush they create a good lather very quickly and with little effort. They've given me consistent and satisfying lathers every time.

Soaps

Shaving soaps are just what the name says, it's a soap
that's made for shaving. It comes in bar or puck form,
and generally lasts for about three months (some
varieties last much longer). They are different from
normal bar soap, though I've heard stories of some
people using regular bar soap also. My experience
with them has been that they take a bit more practice
to master, and a little more time to mix. Both my best
and my worst have been from soaps, with some
absolutely great and others down right terrible, which
I suspect to be a user issue.

Do they actually do a better job protecting your skin than gels or aerosol creams?

I honestly don't know, but I have no reason to think
they are any worse. That said, they absolutely make
for a more enjoyable shaving experience and it's
become a much anticipated part of my shaving ritual.
Preparing and loading the brush, mixing the to your
desire, and getting a fresh, warm lather is incredibly
refreshing. Plus, they have much richer, deeper scents
that not only make for a pleasant shave, but which
also linger on the skin well afterward.

Of the two, I personally lean towards shaving soap.
That being said, I'm primarily using a shaving cream
right now and having a very enjoyable experience.
Luckily, with good soaps costing only a few dollars
and creams not much more, there's no reason that
you only have to choose one!

Razor Blade Review: Treet Platinum

April 6, 2014

I think that it is pronounced like "treat."

When my razor blade pack arrived in the mail I'd heard of most of the varieties already. That's a large part of why it beat out other samplers, it provided some degree of familiarity (if just in name, as I'd only used the Derby blades). While I hadn't heard of ever variety, such as the Sharpedge, I at least knew of their manufacturer, Gillette. There was only one brand, in fact, that I hadn't heard of: Treet. That hasn't stopped them from making quite a name for themselves in the last two weeks of my use.

For many years Treet was known for making carbon steel blades. While these were popular with many for their ability to hold and edge both sharper and longer than stainless steel, they were more prone to rust and thus required more attention.

The industry now primarily manufactures stainless for ease of use, and Treet has followed suit. Made in Pakistan, the Treet Platinum is perhaps not as visible as some other razor blade brands. But if you're looking for a great blade that consistently holds an edge, then this one is right up your ally.

Performance wise, I've found the Tweet Platinum to be comparable to the Shark line of blades. For as close as the Shark Stainless and the Shark Chrome were, the Treet feels like it falls somewhere in the middle: not quite as sharp as the Stainless, but more forgiving; not quite as forgiving as the Chrome, but sharper.

I've found it to give excellent shaves that are so close that it actually makes daily shaving a bit uncertain, giving the hair little time to grow out. To accommodate this, I've found it helpful to alternate morning between two passes (one with the grain and one against) and just one (against the grain). It seems to allow growth to recover enough to provide better shaves than just trying to go as close as possible each time.

Where it is most different is that the Treet seems to hold it's edge much better than most, perhaps better than any other blade I've yet used. While there was certainly some degree of wear, the blade remained sharp and consistent through a full week of shaving. That sharpness and even wear allowed for consistent shaves throughout the week, without the feeling that the blade had substantially changed from when I started. While they are no longer carbon steel (at least, not these ones), the Treet reputation remains intact.

I did notice that the blades seem to be a touch harder to clean. Normally a quick rinse under hot water will get most blades clean, the Treet seemed to hold on to hair and lather a bit more tightly. It only took an extra moment under the water to break it loose, but it was noticeable given how easily other blades rinse.

This may not be the blade's fault though, as I switched to a new shaving cream at the same time I started using the blades, so that may be an issue of the cream just not dissolving in water as easily as my previous shaving soap. It's something to keep an eye on as I use other blades.

Verdict: I've found the Treet blades to be extremely satisfying, and one of the best day to day blades I've used. Others have gotten shaves that feel closer, felt better, etc. But few if any have delivered such great results so consistently. The shave smoothly, they shave well, and they stay sharp, it's hard to ask for more.

Morning Shave: Kicking Spring Off Right

April 13, 2014

After a long, snowy winter spring seems to have finally arrived in Virginia. After a week of blooming the blossoms are starting to fall off the trees, giving way to vibrant green leaves and sprouts. The weather has been gorgeous, cool enough for a light jacket or hoodie in the morning but mid-seventies by the afternoon. Things are looking nice.

So nice in fact, that we haven't turned on the heater or air conditioner in at least a week. Last night we left the windows open, and this morning were treated to a nice, cool home with the sounds of birds outside. And traffic, but hey, you take what you can get.

I've been using Proraso heavily lately as my Col. Conk's shave soap is nearly worn through the puck, but I thought this morning called for a change. Lathering up I was treated to the refreshing scent of bayrum, something I've grown to love. I prefer Col. Conk's to Proraso, while it takes slightly longer to mix the result is a thicker, silkier, longer lasting lather. With a new Feather razor blade two passes and a splash of spice aftershave left me feeling great.

 The shave wasn't quite as close as it might have been, I decided to experiment some with the blade angle and the change just wasn't as good as the previous angle had been getting. Good to know, it'll be helpful for future shaves.

Now I'm enjoying a quiet Sunday morning with my feet kicked up, spending time with my best friend before she heads to Utah to help with her sister's wedding. Life is good.

Razor Blade Review: Feather Hi-Stainless

April 17, 2014

No other razor blade comes with a reputation like the Feather. Universally considered one of the sharpest razor blades available, these Japanese blades have the largest and strongest fan base of any other I've seen. I've yet to see a discussion of favorite or best blades where it wasn't mentioned.

Some people, mistakenly thinking that sharper must mean "better", jump right to the Feather when they first start shaving. But just because a blade is sharp doesn't mean it will work for you, and if you don't have the basics down then it can be a recipe for an unintended bloodletting.

I decided at the outset of the experiment to try and avoid that, and so I saved the Feathers for last. I'm happy to report that during the testing there were no nicks or even significant blood from shaving too close. And I've come to a simple conclusion: these blades rock.

In fact, as I'm anticipating beginning the second round of testing, I'm starting to think that several of my beliefs about other blades may have been mistaken.

With a number of blades I found that they would give me a good, close shave. But, after a day or two shaving closely, I'd have to back off a bit and let things recover otherwise the shave quality would drop slightly. I assumed this was because my hair just wasn't growing back fast enough, and the close shaves over several days would build up some slight irritation from getting more skin than hair.

During my tests with the Feathers I've been shaving as close as I have before, and more consistently. The last few days I've even been going from my normal two passes to three (first with the grain, second across, then finally against the grain). To my surprise and satisfaction, even that slight irritation seems to have gone away.

I have a couple theories on why that might be:

1) It was a result of inexperience or bad technique, which I have improved through practice.

2) Whether because of sharpness or smoothness, Feathers work extraordinary well for me.

Either way, these last couple weeks have been some great shaves.

The one downside I noticed is that by the end of the week I was definitely noticing the blade beginning to dull. Of course, this can be solved simply: either shave less or change the blade more frequently. But, nonetheless, it is the one downside to the blade that I noticed, especially coming off having just been using the Tweet blades that seemingly shaved forever without losing their edge.

But, that complaint is small potatoes. The Feathers are excellent blades, and for quality of shave they've moved to the top of my list.

Very slick.

Shaving on the Fly: Brushing Up For a Family Wedding

April 22, 2014

Using a safety razor is a lot of fun, but if I've found one downside it's that it can be a bit of a hassle to travel with. Last week was my sister-in-law's wedding, held out west where the rest of our family lives, and so my wife and I trekked 2,000 miles across the country to support them. Of course, a wedding means there's going to be ceremony and photos, so that meant I'd need to be shaving.

Unlike a cartridge razor that you can just toss into a backpack or toiletry case, a double-edge razor requires planning ahead. As I discussed previously, the TSA doesn't like loose razor blades in carry-on luggage so I packed a Feather blade in my wife's checked baggage when she flew out (she went early to help get things ready for the occasion).

But that still the question of how to lather up. When I traveled for Christmas I simply brought a small travel can of Barbasol. But this time I decided to make it more interesting. First, I needed to get a brush out there without it getting damaged. I came up with two options:

If I needed to I could use an old paper tube (paper towels or toilet paper) to keep the bristles protected. This wasn't my ideal choice, as the brush could slip and slide around, and the paper (and the brush within) could easily be crushed.

The second option was a prescription bottle. I'd seen it suggested somewhere online (I don't remember where, else I'd give credit), but I didn't have any on hand. So I just went down to the local CVS and asked them for one (a request I'm guessing they don't get often given their confusion at it). I'd planned on paying for them, I figured there might be medicine bottles as a retail item, but they kindly just gave me one for free from the pharmacy. It worked perfectly! The brush was well protected, and it kept the bristles protected throughout the trip (just make sure it's dry before you put it in). The bottle is a bit tall, but the width was perfect and the brush was just fine.

The next question was whether to bring shaving soap or shaving cream. I decided to go with the shaving soap because it's lighter, harder, and dryer. This allowed me to just wrap the soap in a paper towel and stow it along with the rest of my toiletries. Since it's a solid there's no problem getting it through TSA, and since I enjoy it more than my shaving cream it made the travel shave a bit more enjoyable. The only downside is that after months of faithful use, my soap has finally worn through. I can still use it, but it looks like a hula-hoop and its life is definitely on the downhill.

The shaves I got while out there weren't my best. Traveling throws off my rhythm and I just couldn't seem to get as close and even a shave as I'm used to. But they were still enjoyable, and perfectly good for pictures and festivities. It was a beautiful ceremony and reception for a great couple, and wonderful weather.

Flying back security x-rayed my bag, then a second time, before finally placing my razor in a bin by itself and x-raying that. Finally satisfied, they let us through and we headed home. A great trip!

Review: Derby Extra

April 25, 2014

For many wet shavers, Derby is the first razor blade they'll experience.

In the world of double-edge razors, Derby is the McDonalds. They are everywhere, they are cheap, and I haven't seen a lot of people willing to say they like them.

Derby was the razor that I started safety razor shaving with. When I purchased my razor the company included a pack of five Derby blades, and I thought they were wonderful. In fact, I was so impressed with them that I considered just sticking with them rather than seeing what else was out there.

But where's the fun in that?

It's now four months later, I've tried out half a dozen other brands and I decided to go back and see how Derby holds up.

Coming off of shaving with a Feather blade, Derby feels noticeably dull, or at least not as sharp as I remember them feeling. They also seemed to lose their edge faster than I remember, by Friday there was noticeably more effort and attention necessary to get a good shave.

But while I've found razors that do almost everything better than the Derby...I like them.

With a little experience under your belt they are about impossible to cut yourself with (which means I'll probably cut myself the next time I use them). Using a three pass method you can get a pretty good shave with them (definitely not the closest I've gotten, but not bad at all).

And, of all the razors I've gotten, they give the best next day scruff. Don't ask me how, but it's a nice, even, rough stubble that feels great.

Like I said, Derby is the McDonalds of the safety razor world. And you know what, I like McDonalds sometimes. Is it great? Nope. But does it satisfy in its own way?

Yes it does.

Blood! ...My First Use of a Styptic Pencil

April 27, 2014

It was bound to happen sooner or later, really just a matter of time, but today marked my first cut significant enough to warrant a styptic pencil.

First, what is that? A styptic pencil is used to stop bleeding, made up primarily of aluminum sulfate it basically contracts the skin and blood vessels while helping things clot. It has the look and feel of a piece of chalk, with a pointed end to help target the bleeding spot.

I'm not entirely sure what happened, but I think I might have had a pimple or bug bite lurking beneath the two days growth of stubble. I was shaving along on the first pass (with the grain), when I felt a noticeable bump along the back of right jaw. I turned my head to look, and sure enough there was a noticeable amount of blood welling up already.

This probably should have been my cue to leave the area alone. Being the wise man that I am, I just went ahead lathering and shaving it twice more (across the grain and against the grain). Each time I'd wash my face, apply shaving cream, and in a moment have a nice red blotch appear in the white foam. Is that the best way to handle a bleeder? Probably not, but meh.

I wrapped up the shave and gave a cold water wash, which normally handles anything bleeding. There was still a bit of blood coming out, not much but enough that I decided that I both wanted to avoid getting it on my church clothes and that this would be a great time to try out my styptic pencil. It'd been sitting on my counter for six months doing nothing, might as well see how it worked.

Everything I'd heard is that it would burn. Honestly, I didn't fell anything. I pressed it against the cut, which wasn't large at all for the amount of blood that had come out, and after about ten seconds pulled it back away. No more blood, cut hardly noticeable. (comma) and except for some white residue that appeared a moment later no problems.

I'm sold. If you're thinking of getting into wet shaving, or you're already trying it yourself, pick yourself up a styptic (an alum bloc also works I'm told). Did I NEED it? Maybe not, but it sure was handy.

Review II: Astra Superior Platinum

May 7, 2014

Normally my reviews come out on Thursday or Friday. That's when my razor blades are ready to change and so it makes sense to wrap things up all at once. This one is a bit early because the result is abundantly clear: I'm just not a fan.

In my previous review I wasn't thrilled about them. In fact, they were the only blades I used where I wasn't looking forward to shaving. The last two weeks have been more of the same.

Performance wise they actually aren't bad. With either two passes or three they got a reasonably close shave. The blades hold an edge well, and shaving five times a week they were still feeling sharp by the end of it. While the shaves never felt as close and as smooth as what some of my preferred razors provide, they were just fine for work, school, or church.

So why don't I like them?

For starters, the shaves just didn't feel great. While they looked fine and felt close, they didn't leave my face feeling as clean and groomed as what I like. The only two major nicks I've gotten have both been from Astra blades. And, while I can't exactly explain how, shaving with them just isn't as much fun.

I know a lot of people love them, and if they work well for them then great. But they're just not for me. I've used them for four weeks and that was enough, I gave away my last Astra blade a couple days ago.

Maybe someday I'll change my mind about them, but for now I remain unimpressed.

The Rise of the 3 Pass Shave

May 11, 2014

For years while I used a cartridge razor I would only make one pass while shaving: against the grain. It was quick, it was simple, and it got the job done.

Since switching to a safety razor I have almost completely abandoned that method. If I'm really rushing I might try it, but for day to day shaving I largely adopted a two pass method: lather, shave with the grain, lather again (with what remains on the brush), shave against the grain.

This has been my daily routine shave for months. Starting in April, however, things began to change. Right around the time I was testing the Feather blades I decided to try out using a three pass method, which I had seen numerous blogs and websites recommend.

The method is simple: lather, shave with the grain (WTG), lather, shave across the grain at a right angle (XTG), lather, shave against the grain (then shave against the grain) (ATG). You can reload your brush for lathers, or you can just load it once if the soap will last you all three lathers. When shaving across the grain, I start at the ear/ sideburn and shave toward the nose, then work my way down the neck, leaving the mustache area for last.

It's taken some getting used to, but it is slowly replacing my two pass method of shaving. I still use two passes for more daily shaving. It saves a bit on time, and gives a very nice shave. But for special days, like Sundays, date night, etc. I'm using three passes almost exclusively. It leaves my face just a bit smoother, gives a more even shave (perhaps simply because the extra pass is another chance to catch stray hairs), and the shave lasts noticeably longer.

And if you're enjoying shaving, it gives you a few more minutes before you start the day, something I won't complain about!

Save Your Soap: Melting Old Soap Into a New Puck

May 15, 2014

For Christmas my wife bought me a puck of Col. Conk's Bayrum shaving soap. Unlike shaving cream, shaving soap looks much like a regular, round bar of soap. Specially made to create a good, protecting lather, I prefer it to shaving cream and have enjoyed using it for the last five months.

Unfortunately all that use takes a toll. When using a brush to create a shaving lather you first "load" the brush, which means getting condensed soap into the bristles to then put onto your face. Due to a combination of brush shape and my natural tendency to load from the middle of the bar, what started as a bar about one inch thick was eventually worn down to a soap donut.

This created a problem for lathering. When loading a brush soap naturally congregates in the middle of the bristles, so having soap without a middle means that it is very difficult to load the brush properly. The result is a thinner lather that does not last long either on the brush or face.

After a bit of internet research I came across a solution: melting. While it does not work for all soaps (such as triple-milled and I think also soaps that are tallow based), for others you can heat the soap to a melting point, then reform it into a new shape.

To do this I put mine in a small, microwave safe glass bowl (my wife was very supportive of microwaving soap in her dishes). I'd heard some say to start with 5 seconds, others said 30. I went with 10 seconds to start then checked it to see if more was needed. To my delight, the soap had completely melted (and was smelling great!).

After letting it cool the result was a solid block of soap, evenly thick and perfectly smooth. While I could have tried to get it out of the dish, I decided just to leave it in until I use it up (or we need the dish). If I needed to get it out I might try floating the dish in warm water to soften the portion touching glass, but we'll cross that bridge later.

I tried it out this morning, which also meant that I was trying out lathering soap in a bowl for the first time. I've always just lathered on my hand or directly on my face, so I was interested to see what the result would be.

It worked great.

Melting the soap gave it a nice smooth surface. Before loading I soaked the brush in warm water, and spread a few drops of warm water on the top of the soap to soften things up. With about 10-15 seconds of swirling I had a brush loaded thick and ready for application.

The bowl really helped to get the soap into the brush. Both the first and second application were far thicker than usual creating a smooth, protecting lather. I expected the soap to be running low by this point, but going into the third pass the brush was still loaded heavily with soap. It's like the Energizer bunny of shaving.

The result was probably the best lather I've ever had, from the beginning to the end of shaving. It was so successful that once I find a permanent shaving bowl I might just try melting soap directly into it from the start rather than waiting for it to be worn down through use.

And to think I was contemplating just chucking the left over soap and getting a new bar. What a waste that would have been!

How My Shave
Hobby Developed

May 20, 2104

When I first began looking into getting a safety razor, it took all of five minutes to realize that there was more than just a hobby base surrounding it. There's an entire sub-culture. Ok, that might be a bit extreme, but that's sure what it looked like to my novice eye.

That there existed dedicated hobbyists to shaving seemed bizarre to me. It's shaving, that thing you do in the morning because you have to. Why would anyone make that their hobby? I resolved to myself that while I might get a razor, I was not adopting a lifestyle.

What I didn't realize at the time was that I was hobby starved. For years, since I was a kid, my hobby was computers and video games. When I hit college I picked up firearms, enjoying the mechanics, camaraderie, and skill required. But these pursuits got hit hard the last few years for a couple reasons.

First, I just didn't have the time. I got into law school and then got married after my first semester, and so what little free time I had away from work and school was reserved for family and church. While my wife is extremely supportive of both hobbies, I just didn't have the time to dedicate to them like I used to (especially since my preferred range is half an hour away).

Second, I just can't afford them like I used to. With the costs of books, a family, and tuition, I can't afford a good gaming system. Similarly, the massive gun and ammo runs that have occurred following Pres. Obama's elections have driven prices sky high in the shooting world (though they are beginning to drop some).

I had been priced out of my hobbies, both in costs to time and money.

However, at the same time it also created a fertile field for shaving. My initial efforts, meant to save me money, inadvertently laid the groundwork for a new hobby: research, involvement, and commitment. When my wife gave me a brush and shaving soap for Christmas the foundations were in place, and things advanced rapidly.

What made this different from my other hobbies, and substantially more maintainable on a student budget and schedule, were the same things that had been the previous undoing. The additional time commitment was minimal. I was already shaving every day for work, so the change meant just a few extra minutes in the morning. I could afford to be involved in it every day if I wanted, with barely a noticeable change to my existing schedule. And, were I to stick to the basics, the hobby would actually save me money over how I was previously shaving, and is cheaper to pursue than either videogames or shooting. For the cost of the ammunition I would use for one day of shooting I can have buy months' worth of soap, blades, or aftershaves.

And so, contrary to what I expected when I began, I have witnessed myself fall headlong into the shaving hobby. Though my collection is small, I have numerous blades, two kinds of soaps, and two kinds of aftershaves, with many others I would like to try.

I still love video games, and I still love shooting. I look forward to when I can do them more often. But I'm glad to have found a new pastime in the interim.

Review: Proraso (Green) Shaving Cream

May 22, 2014

I thought "sapone" was the scent…turns out it's Italian for "soap."

Several months back I asked around about what soaps I should try out, and the name that came up the most was Proraso.

Proraso is an Italian shaving cream, sold in either a tub or tube (like toothpaste). It comes in three varieties, green, white, and red, with white and green being the most common. I decided to pick up a tub of green, which is the standard formula. I'd never tried a shaving cream that you mix before, and I was excited to see how well it worked (plus, I'd heard the tub was really useful for travel and mixing once the soap had run out).

I've been using it for two months now and I'm happy to say that this stuff is great.

Mixing it is similar to mixing up a shaving soap. You wet the brush, load the soap onto the bristles for 20-30 seconds, and then mix up a lather however you prefer. Personally, I apply directly to the face and I've found a good loading is plenty for three applications plus extra.

The first thing I noticed was the smell, which I believe is eucalyptus. It was strong and eye opening, much different than the bay rum I was used to. The second thing I noticed was the sensation: this stuff makes your skin tingle. The best I can describe it is it's like having wet skin with a cool breeze. Not enough to make you cold, but to make you feel crisp. I notice it a little bit on application, but really feel it as the skin is exposed through shaving. This sensation fades some with daily use, but alternating with other soaps means that it's more noticeable on days you use it.

The cream provides good protection, even with thin applications. It also applies much more evenly than I've gotten with shaving soap.

There are a couple downsides to Proraso. First, it can be a bit tricky to get the right mixture of water. Too much and it's runny, too little and it will dry out on your face before you can get to it. Second, it is stickier on the razor blade, so it takes more effort to clean the blade of soap and hair. Finally, it seems to leave a dusting of soap particles on hard to reach places of the razor, even with a good washing after use.

But these haven't stopped me from enjoying it thoroughly. With practice the mixture gets more consistent, with warm water the soap and hair cleans easily enough, and a weekly in depth cleaning of the razor when you change the blade keeps everything in order.

Once I run out I will be hard pressed not to run back out and buy more, it's great stuff and I highly recommend it.

Review II: Personna Platinum Chrome

May 25, 2014

When I first reviewed the Personna Platinum Chromes I remember noting how sharp they were. Since then I've used other blades that feel sharper to me, so I was interested in how I'd like these now that I have more experience under my belt.

First the good things: these blades hold up. While the first week was a bit slower, I've been using three pass shaves for all seven days a week of the last week and the blade did great. With a new blade on Sunday by the time Saturday came around I wasn't noticing pulling or tugging associated with a dulling blade. Keeping the stubble short might have helped that, though I would think that the additional passes would have taken a toll. But they held up well until the end.

Second, while they aren't the sharpest blade around they feel like a good middle ground. The sharpest razor doesn't always work best for everyone, they aren't a one size fit all item. Rather, you should try to find the sharpest blade that works for you, regardless of where it falls on the spectrum. The Personna fits well in the middle.

Finally, enjoy them. Are they my favorite to shave with? No, but unlike the Astra (which shaved decently but which I just didn't enjoy) despite any shave shortcomings I didn't find myself frustrated or disliking the experience.

There were two downsides I noticed to these blades:

First, for the life of me I just couldn't seem to get a consistent shave out of them. Some days would be close, others would be rough; some parts of my face would be smooth, the same part on the other side would be alright. I just can't seem to get an even shave day to day with them.

Second, while I did like them, other blades just feel more fun. That may be an odd way to describe razor blades, but I just enjoy shaving with other blades more. While two blades might get you to the same goal, it seems silly not to notice which one gives you a better experience while getting there. The Personnas do a good job, and I don't dislike them, but I just like others more.

But as I said above, they are good blades. I enjoyed using them, they hold up well, and give a workable shave for day to day use.

3 Pass Shave v. 3 Blade Razor

May 27, 2014

I was recently asked the question: if I use a Mach3 razor, is that the same as doing a three pass shave?

The answer is no, but it's a good question. Another time I might do an actual result comparison by doing by, but for now I'm just going to explain the difference. For those unaware, this is a Mach3 razor has three blades mounted in succession, the idea of which is to give you tree cuts at the hair with one pass. It's understandable why one might think this means that one pass is the same as three passes with a safety razor. But it's not.

The primary difference is that a Mach3 cuts the hair in the same direction with each blade, while a three pass technique with double-edge (DE) safety razor is generally considered to involve one pass with the grain, one pass across the grain, and one pass against the grain.

Why is this important?

When a razor connects with a hair the hair resists. When you shave with the grain the hair has more opportunity to bend when pressed by the razor, which reduces the closeness of the shave. By gradually increasing the hair's natural resistance to the blade by moving across and then against the grain, while at the same time reducing the hair's length with each pass, it allows you shave optimally against the hair on the final pass while reducing the likelihood of irritation, unevenness, or other problems associated with shaving against the grain outright.

A Mach3 can also be used this way, of course. In fact, pretty much everyone I talk to that uses a multi-blade cartridge ends up making at least two passes with it (one with and one against the grain). However, you are then making just as many passes as with a DE razor, meaning you've now had nine blade passes over the hair.

That's if the later blades are even connecting properly, of course.

The secondary benefits of multiple passes with a DE razor over one pass with Mach3 is that it allows the hair time to recover, while also ensuring that each time your blade is passing it is at a pressure and angle that you desire. If the hair bends while being cut by a Mach3, there simply isn't much time for it to straighten before the second and third blade hit it. But by giving it time while you complete your first pass, lather, than shave up to the location again, you allow more time for the hair to recover, which in turn improves your ability to shave it.

And of course, one of the best benefits of the three pass method with a DE razor is that DE shaving is a lot of fun, and it gives you more opportunity to enjoy it!

So that's the difference. It boils down to the fact that each pass of a three pass technique is intended to be different than the first, while each blade of a Mach3 is supposed to do the same thing as the others. If that works for you, good deal.

Breaking in New Blades

June 1, 2014

Occasionally you realize something that, in hind sight, you should have realized months before. Today was one of those days.

Since I started shaving with a safety razor I assumed that the first day shaving with a new blade would be the best opportunity to shave well with it. That each blade began at optimal sharpness and smoothness, with each subsequent shave degrading the blade.

This morning it hit me like a lightning bolt: like many tools and machines, some blades need to be broken in.

Sunday has always been new blade day, and I figured it would be my best shave. But as I was pondering during this morning's deforestation, I realized that Sunday shaves usually don't feel the best. In fact, its usually not until Monday or Tuesday that the shaves feel closest and most comfortable.

Though this will take more observation, I believe that some blades peak around day two or three before declining on shave quality. While this may seem trivial, figuring this out will mean that if there is a big event to prepare for, such as a wedding, interview, date, etc, prior planning will help provide the highest quality shave by coordinating peak blade condition.

This really should not be as interesting as it is, but I'm kinda geeking out!

Review II: Shark Super Chrome

June 6, 2014

Since the previous couple of razors hadn't felt much different than I remembered the first time I tested them, I expected the Chrome to be the same. I was wrong.

The Shark Super Chrome is the first razor I've retested where things felt noticeably different. The last time I remember thinking it felt much like other razors, but more forgiving. While the latter part remains true, I've found something else the last two weeks: they feel rather dull.

That's not to say that they don't shave well. I've enjoyed ample great shaves with these blades. They shave great out of the box and even better once broken in. But the change from what I remembered was so marked that at first I thought it was just a bad blade. When both behaved similarly, it seems more likely that it's just how they are.

As I said though, they were enjoyable and are very forgiving. My morning shaves have gotten very quick and cavalier, which has the potential to cause problems down the road. But it was something I could get away with the Chrome, and it was fun to back off from slow and deliberate for a couple weeks in exchange for quick and functional.

If you're looking for sharp blades, these are still razors. But you can definitely find sharper out there. But if you're looking for reliable blades that will let you get away with mistakes, these are a great option.

Lasts Gasps of a Dying Soap

June 11, 2014

Col. Conk's bayrum shave soap was the first shaving soap I'd tried. Before that it was either gels or Barbersol, applied with my hands. But after I purchased my double-edge razor my wife got me the soap and a brush as a gift, and I've been loving it ever since.

I wasn't sure that I would. Lather didn't interest me as much as the razor, and I wasn't sure it would be worth the effort.

But what I found was a rich and rewarding experience. My first attempts, in hind sight, were terrible. Then I thought I got the hang of it, and it was fun. In hind sight though, the results here were also terrible. I just didn't know enough to know that yet.

The last couple months have seen a lot of improvement. More foam, thicker and longer lasting lather, better protection. When I wore through the puck, the melted remains in a small dish taught me about the benefits of using a bowl to load.

But the time is far spent, and there is little soap remaining. Probably just a few more shaves at most.

It lasted about 5 1/ 2 months. Not bad. A good soap apparently goes a long way. It also means it may be time to get new soap soon. It's hard not to simply get another puck of Conk's, but I've heard good thing about some of the other brands out there (such as Mama Bears) so I think I will try some out. Experiment.

In the meanwhile, I heartily recommend Col. Conk's Bayrum. I can't speak to their other products, but this one treated me well.

Review: Lucky Tiger
Aftershave & Face Tonic

June 13, 2014

I've never been an aftershave guy, or cologne for that matter.) Growing up I remember my dad having Old Spice in glass bottles (and an elk shaped bottle holder), and occasionally for Christmas I would get a small bottle of some type of cologne, but I'd usually just forget to use it.

When I took up shaving with a double-edge razor I got a bottle of CVS brand spice aftershave. It worked well, and I grew used to the scent, the soft burn, and the feeling of tight skin that would come at the end of a shave.

But as I explored my options with razors, blades, soaps, and creams, questions naturally arose in my mind about what is out there for after the shave.

I first saw Lucky Tiger on a shelf at Grooming Lounge, and the old timey style of the bottle (plastic, made to look like amber glass) and label intrigued me. I got a bottle a month or two later, just as spring has been arriving.

It was a good decision. Lucky Tiger has a crisp orange scent to it, making it a refreshing start to a spring or summer day. I grew up near orange groves, and my grandparents had orange trees in their yard, so it is a familiar and happy smell to me. The scent fads extremely fast, within a few seconds, giving a burst of citrus before going to your natural smell (allowing you to use other colognes if you want, I rarely do).

There is no alcohol, which took some getting used to. Much like mouthwash, I had associated the alcohol burn with the notion that it was doing something. For the first fee days I wasn't sure it actually was doing something, and I almost regretted the purchase.

But I found Lucky Tiger is best appreciated with regular use. It is both an aftershave and a tonic, so it is meant to help keep your skin healthy. It leaves my skin feeling soft and slightly slick for hours afterward. At first I associated this with oily, but I soon realized that its just how my skin uses when I regularly use something designed to moisturize.

I still love the sharpness of alcohol-based aftershaves, and that is probably be what I try next. But Lucky Tiger has earned a spot on my shelf. If you're looking for something to invigorate and close up nicks, this may not be for you. But if you're looking for a smooth and refreshing start, I highly recommend it.

Review II: Gillette 7 O'clock Sharpedge

June 28, 2014

Because Gillette 7 O'clock Sharpedge were stand out blades when I first tested them several months ago, I found myself greatly anticipating using them again.

Much to my surprise I ran into trouble almost immediately.

The blades themselves were what I remembered. Extremely sharp, as the name implies, they cut through stubble quickly and easily. But the results were problematic, after a day of shaving I found myself with sensitive skin that didn't want a close shave.

To solve this problem I adjusted my method. Rather than making one pass with the grain and one against, I switched to one pass with the grain and one across it. This gave me a slightly rougher shave, but the irritation cleared up immediately. After a few days I switched back to with and against the grain, and the irritation didn't return. I suspect the problem was that I got used to using more pressure and aggressive methods with duller blades, which the Sharpedge won't let me get away with.

With the issue resolved I found myself having wonderful shaves throughout the week. Even pushing the blades past their normal week use to ten days gave me decent, though noticeably declining, shaves.

While I have enjoyed many of the blades I've used, these are among the few I am seriously considering buying in bulk. While they aren't very forgiving, they shave excellent for me, and they are simply fun to use. It's hard to define that last category, but some blades just feel boring to me.

These aren't one of them. I am now out of blades, and I'll be keeping my eyes open to pick up more.

Review II: Treet Platinum

July 20, 2014

When I last reviewed the Treet Platinum I had a hard time coming up with things to talk about. Not because it I hadn't been paying attention those weeks, I had. Nor because I was having writers block, because I wasn't.

Rather the Treet Platinum was some a mild razor for me that I didn't know what more to say about it. It was forgiving, gave no irritation, and a thoroughly workable shave. Were I to pick one razor blade for beginners, it would compete with Derby as an excellent place to start.

This round of shaving is little different, I don't know quite what to say about it. While I had slightly more irritation this time the shaves were close and very comfortable. Not the closest shaves, nor the longest lasting. Other blades are simply more fun.

But Treet still has something going for it: consistency. While the good shaves aren't excellent, the bad shaves aren't terrible.

It's a shave you can count on, and a good one at that. It's not a blade I get excited over, but it's both a good and a reliable shave. It's hard to go wrong with that.

Wall Drug: South Dakota Shave Supplies

July 26, 2014

Wall Drug is a small drug store, nestled between Mt. Rushmore and the Badlands National Park. A country stop where I figured I could find some old-fashioned shave goods.

Or, at least that's what I thought. It turns out that Wall Drug, located in Wall, SD (a town whose primary existence, from what I can, is to facilitate the drug store), is a straight up tourist attraction.

According to the menu/ history pamphlet that we were given, Wall Drug was struggling until the owners came up with the idea to offer free ice water to anyone who stopped. Several decades later the store now consists of...well, pretty much everything. Bookstore, restaurant, leather goods, candy shop, giant fiberglass jackalope, an animatronic piano playing monkey, and more gift shops than you can shake a stick at.

And, as it turns out, a small apothecary style shaving shop with a small but quality old fashioned shaving selection.

Most drug stores these days will carry some off brand razor blades, maybe a generic bar of shave soap. To its credit, Wall Drug's stock may have been small, but it was quality goods. There were several Muhle brand razors, which use the same razor head as my Edwin Jagger de89L (the difference is in the handle). There was a number of bowls, and even a couple of scuttles, which is a shaving bowl with a hot water bowl underneath to keep the lather warm.

Finally, they had a full line of Col. Conk's shave supplies, both shaving soap and aftershave. I'm a big fan of Col. Conk's, and with my last bar having been used up a couple weeks before I was already thinking of buying more. Wall Drug's prices, oddly enough for a tourist stop, were quite good.

So I picked up some souvenirs! Amber, Almond, and Bayrum shave soap. They also had Lime, but honestly, Lime smelled kinda funny and I didn't see myself using it.

Wall, SD might be a bit out of your way simply to get some shaving goods, unless of course you already live in south-west South Dakota. But if you're visiting Mt. Rushmore and places east, it might be worth your stop.

And they still have free ice water.

Review II: Shark Super Stainless

August 3, 2014

Eight months ago, as I first began testing different kinds of razor blades, I tried Shark Super Stainless for the first time. Previously I had only ever used Derby blades, which gave me quite a good shave and which I had learned DE safety razor shaving with. Moving on to the Sharks felt like a graduation, and the shaves felt incredible. I seriously considered just ordering a pack of 100 and stopping the test right then.

I have now cycled through the rest of the sampler pack twice over (save the Feathers, which will be tested a second time over the next couple weeks), and I specifically saved the Sharks until last so I could both try them head to head with the Feathers, and so I could test them again with much more experience than the first time.

Alas, how the mighty have fallen.

For the last two weeks my shaves have been disappointing. Inconsistent. Not at all what I remembered them being. Even on the best days the shaves were only good, not great. Most days were average, and there were one or two that really weren't good at all. At the same time the razors seemed to dull quicker than I remembered, making for a rapidly declining experience during the week.

I have several theories on why this might be:

1) User issues. It's possible I'm just not shaving as well as I was eight months ago, and so regardless of the equipment the shaves will be worse. This might be the issue, but seems unlikely. While I might have been in a funk, I don't think I would have gotten so noticeably worse at this.

2) Bad blades. The blades I used before might have simply been better blades, and the ones I used this time weren't as good quality. This also seems unlikely though, as they came out of the same pack. Different packs in a big box? Sure. But to have three good blades, then two bad ones? That raises an eyebrow.

3) My expectations have changed as my experience has gone up, and the novelty of safety razor shaving has gone down. That's not to say I dislike shaving like this, quite the opposite. But as I've grown more accustomed to it the perhaps now I'm not as willing to overlook some things, and take more notice of others. With other razors to compare it to, perhaps now they don't seem as special.

I'm leaning toward #3, as you can probably tell from how I discounted the other two but not that one. Whatever the reason though, the Shark Stainless just didn't do it for me this time. I'm disappointed about that, I really liked them and also happened to think the packaging was entertaining.

But that's the way these things go. Perhaps I'll swing back toward them in time. Maybe I love them in winter, but not in summer. Who knows? In the meanwhile I'll keep looking, and maybe our paths will cross again.

Cold Water Shave: That's Brisk

August 11, 2014

Many shave guides extol the warm water shave as the only way to go, and admittedly, I normally use warm water as well. But today I was feeling like something a little different, something cool and crisp after my morning run and for a warm summer day.

Lathered with warm water like normal, using Proraso soap. Proraso has a cool tingle to it to begin with, and I thought it would go well with the cold shave. I ran the Feather blade in my razor under cold water, and got to work.

The cold metal combined with the Proraso was a great combination, once the air hit a newly shaved spot it felt like an autumn morning. I'd run the razor under warm water to break up the soap, then once clean I'd run it back under cold to get it ready for skin.

Two passes left me feeling great, then some spice aftershave to give a warming kicker. Perfect.

Headed into work now feeling great, smooth face and no irritation.

Review II: Feather Hi-Stainless

August 17, 2014

When I first tried Feather razor blades I was nervous. They came with a reputation for sharpness, and are considered one of the best blades you can buy. I hadn't had any major shaving incidents, and I didn't want to start. But they impressed me so much, and gave a shave so enjoyable, that they were probably the best I'd used thus far. With this second round of testing, and with some blades that I remembered loving suddenly falling short, I was again nervous, this time that a blade I thought so highly of wouldn't live up to what I remembered.

To its credit, Feather didn't disappoint.

Once again I found myself enjoying closer shaves and with less irritation than I have in weeks. Whether two day growth or daily shaves for work, it did its job well. So well in fact, that as I begin to look for new blade sampler packs to try it is one of only a couple blades that I'm planning to keep on hand.

The other blade? Derby, oddly enough.

That's something I don't understand. Feather is considered one of the sharpest blades out there, best for once you know what you're doing, while Derby is often seen as a starter blade. A great start for new shavers. Yet these two are perhaps the only two that haven't disappointed me yet.

I don't know why this is, but I do know that I like them. Feather has treated me well, I'm loving the work it does, and it will have a spot in my shave supplies for a long time to come.

After Action Report: The Great Shave Experiment

August 18, 2014

On Friday of last week an eight month experiment came to an official end: I had used each of the razors in my sampler pack for at least four weeks, and tracked my experience through dozens of written posts.

Along the way I've learned a lot, some of which is particular to what works for me, and some that would benefit anyone. Tiny refinements have been made, as well as major changes (for example, I started using one side of the razor on one day, switching sides with each day so, whereas now I use both sides during a shave so that the wear is more even).

And yet, it's not really over.

Now would be a great time to walk away from things. I'll keep shaving of course, but having set out with a goal that has now been accomplished it would be easy to declare success and perhaps turn my energy elsewhere.

But I'm having too much fun to do that, so instead I'm going to keep going until I lose interest or time to keep it up. Because why not? I still have to shave, I'm still going to be using a double-edge razor, and I'll still be looking for new and enjoyable shave supplies. Might as well document it for the fine folk of the Internet.

Shaving Fail: A Harsh Lesson in Grain

August 25, 2014

Whenever I see old pictures or movies about pre-Wright brothers flying machines, usually some bizarre creation that seems to have no chance of working, I wonder to myself, "what were they thinking?" Of course the answer is simple, they were thinking it would work. Having grown up knowing what airplanes, helicopters, and rockets look like I have information that they didn't. What they had was what they thought was a good idea, right up to the time that they decided to try it out.

The other week I had a good idea.

Why, I asked myself, when shaving across the grain, do I always start at the ear and go toward the chin? What if I started at the chin, and shaved toward the neck? Perhaps all this time I've been missing out on an ideal shave technique, getting closer shave with less irritation!

I owed it to myself to try, so one morning I lathered up and when it came time to shave across the grain I put metal to skin and gave it a try.

The results were instantly terrible. I could feel the blade gripping and pulling, a rough uneven resistance coming from my skin. With trepidation I finished the side, and with blood already beginning to form the experiment was called off nearly as soon as it had begun.

So, I will no longer be shaving in the direction of my chin to my ear. I don't have to learn that lesson twice!

Getting Myself a Shave Bowl

August 31, 2014

One of the first things I thought when I started DE wet shaving was that I needed to pick up a shaving bowl. I had no idea what they did or how they worked, but it seemed like something I would need...I guess.

Subsequently, that was one of the first misconceptions about wet shaving that I found myself corrected on. As it turns out, a shaving bowl isn't necessary at all.

For months I simply lathered directly on my hand or face. It wasn't until I had worked my way through my first shave soap puck and needed to melt it down that I got around to actually trying a bowl out. What I found was that while I wasn't using it for building lather, it did help significantly with loading the brush with soap. So when it came time to get more soap I decided to find myself a bowl (my wife, ever patient with my commandeering the dishware, gently requested that I find an alternative container).

Shaving bowls can run for $10-15 or more online, but being cheap I had no desire to pay that much. Instead, I hit up Wal-Mart and got a cereal bowl for a dollar.

Is it specially intended for shaving? No, but it fits perfectly in my hand, is a great depth and width for a brush, and oh yes, it costs a dollar.

I've never used shaving cream from a tube, which is usually then mixed in a bowl before application. Nor do I use a bowl much for lathering, as I mentioned. So what do I use the shave bowl for? Loading the brush, which is getting the soap into the brush and bristles so that when you try and lather you have something to work with, is one of the most important steps in a good shave. You can load directly off a free standing block of soap, and I did so for many months. But I've found a bowl to be helpful, and so that's what I decided to use it for.

First I molded the soap into the bowl. The most universal method of this is, from what I am told, using a hand cranked grater to shred the soap, then packing it by hand. However, if you know that the soap can be melted in a microwave (not all can or should) then you can save yourself a lot of time. I decided to use Col. Conk's Almond soap, I've melted their Bayrum scented soap before without problem so I assumed that the Almond would work just as well.

Step 1: Put soap in the bowl.

Once the soap is in the bowl I used short bursts in the microwave to soften and melt the soap without cooking or bubbling it. Eventually, in a minute or two, it liquefied. You don't have to cool it off, it does that on it's own, but I decided to put it in a bowl of cool water to help speed things up.

Once it cooled I had a full puck's worth of soap in the bowl, ready for use. Having used it for several weeks now, I can report that the bowl has been working great! While a specialty bowl might bring some additional benefits, and melting it into the bowl means that until I use all of the soap the bowl is tied up (reducing its use if I feel like more soap variety), the low cost and ease of acquiring (as opposed to ordering online) makes it a welcome investment and tool in my growing shaving kit.

Safety Razor Safety: Disposing of Old Blades

September 9, 2014

Safety razors are, as the name suggests, actually incredibly safe. One of my biggest worries when I started shaving with a DE razor, and the biggest concern I hear from others, is that using an old fashioned razor will turn into some kind of Sweeny Todd nightmare (I've not actually seen the movie, but I have a good idea what happens). But the razor has the name for a reason, it is designed to protect you from the razor blade.

All that changes when it's time to change the blade. The guards come off, and you have to handle the blade on your own. This, again, isn't actually a big deal. If you're careful to avoid touching the razor's edge you'll be fine, and I've yet to cut myself at all changing them. But you're left with a used razor blade, which is still extremely sharp, that now needs to be disposed of. You could of course just put it in the garbage. But this risks the blade cutting through the bag, making a mess, and possibly cutting you or the garbage man when the trash is taken out.

There are several ways to avoid this. First, some blades are sold in plastic containers which include a blade disposal slot on the bottom. New blades come out the top, old blades go in the bottom. However many blades are sold in paper containers that simply hold the new blades, so this isn't always an option.

Any choice you might have, if you live in an older home, is a razor blade disposal slot. While no longer in style, some older homes included a small slot in the medicine cabinet that you simply dropped the blade into, like a coin in a vending machine. It opened into the empty space of your wall, and since the blades are so thin it might take years or decades to fill.

But most people don't have that as an option. For a similar result you can use what's called a blade bank. The idea is simple: a hard plastic shell with a small slot for the blade, which allows the blades to be collected and handled without any risk of accidentally cutting anything or anyone. Once it's full you simply throw it away.

This is the method I use, though I didn't want to buy one (I have heard that some stores include a blade bank with razor blade purchases, but I have not encountered that yet). Instead, I use a small flavored butter jar, the kind that looks like a small mason jar. Once it's full, into the garbage or recycling it will go, and no one is at risk of getting hurt.

Cold Water Proraso: How Water Temperature Changes the Shave Experience

September 14, 2014

There is widespread consensus among wet shavers that hot water provides the best shave. Nearly every shaving guide I've read recommends it, mostly with some claim of superior performance because of how the hot water softens your skin and stubble. There are, of course, some who disagree with this and are instead ardent advocates of cold water shaving.

I enjoy both, and I'm not going to argue that someone gives up one for the other. But while both have always appealed to me for various reasons, this summer I've discovered that Proraso soap makes for an excellent cold water experience.

I discovered this one day after a long morning run. It was hot outside, I was trying to cool down before I headed to work, and a warm water shave just didn't sound very appealing. So I lathered up with as cold of water as I could get, and went to shaving.

The result was wonderful. A hot shave with Proraso creates a sauna like soothing, both in feel and smell. But by shaving cold when I was already warm the normal tingles and sharp smell created a chilling effect, much like when you step outside on a cold day and feel the air crisp your skin and chill your nose with each breath. By the time I finished my face was smooth and cold feeling, a sharp contrast with how I started, and with a splash of spice aftershave it felt almost holiday like. It was one of the most refreshing shaves I've ever had.

The cold water did have some draw backs. It thickened the soap, (remove) so when I needed to clean the blade of stubble I'd have to run it under hot water to break up the gunk, then back under cold to chill the now clean blade for the next pass. But, with modern indoor plumbing this really wasn't a problem at all. By being cold it also made it more difficult to lather, again because of thicker soap. A bit more water than usual did the trick on that part.

Whichever works best for you, do it. But how to use cold water to change the experience is a trick I'm slowly working to build. And if I ever have to shave away from hot water, at least I'll be used to it!

A Closer Look at the Mach3: Going Back After DE Shaving

September 22, 2014

I've said from the start that I didn't switch to double-edge (DE) shaving from a cartridge razor because I was unhappy with the shaves I was getting. For me, the switch was almost entirely about money, and a little bit about the "cool" factor. This week I ordered six new brands of razor blades, sort of a do-it-yourself sampler pack I cobbled together, and though it's most expensive to order them in small quantities rather than a bulk purchase of a single brand I still only paid $15 for about 30 weeks worth of razors. Not too shabby.

Since it will take a few days for them to arrive, it seemed like a good opportunity to do something I've been wanting to do for a few months: try out the Mach3.

This seems a bit silly on it's face because I've used one for over a decade (with a Fusion thrown in here or there). What don't I know? The answer is that while, yes, I've got years of experience using one I've never had anything to compare it to. Things are different now, so this week I'm using a cartridge razor again (luckily I had one laying around for the last ten or eleven months).

There likely will not be an official review of it, though I may do so if I feel so inclined. Rather the point has been to remind myself what it is like, so I can draw better comparisons when people ask me about the difference. Thus far I've noticed several things:

It feels light and cheap. I've grown used to a heavier, metal razor. Going back to plastic just feels weird and flimsy.

It's not much of a time saver. The prep time remains the same, the type of razor you're using doesn't change whether you're using foam from a can or mixing your own lather. Actually shaving is slightly quicker, but making two passes the time difference is probably only a few minutes at most.

It's easier to miss spots. The cartridge doesn't seem as effective at removing lather, leaving a good amount of watery slop, which makes it difficult to see spots you've missed. Consequently, I ended up missing spots that I normally (but not always) get with a DE blade.

The shave is less consistent than I remember. Some spots get wonderfully smooth, primarily my cheeks and mustache area. But my neck and chin, where there is more definition, are a toss up. Parts are smooth, others have a fair amount of stubble remaining even after a two pass shave. It's not a bad shave, it's perfectly suitable for a day, but it is by no means great.

Finally, it just doesn't feel as good. The shave itself is dull and simple, while the stubble that's left and whiskers that grow back feel...weird. Whereas DE shaving results in a scruff that feels like good sandpaper, the Mach3 results in a pokey, inconsistent sharpness. It's not uncomfortable, but it's noticeably different and not in a good way.

My thoughts thus far are decidedly "eh." While I didn't switch to DE shaving because I was unhappy with the shave or the experience I was getting from a cartridge, those seeds have now been planted. Having been where the grass is both greener and cheaper (though admittedly more difficult to get to, simply because few grocery or drug stores carry the items in any variety, if at all), I'm simply not impressed with the results I'm getting. I'll certainly use cartridges in the future, they do have some advantages and I don't hate them. Plus, there's a heck of a lot of variety out there so maybe some other brands or models are better.

But I now have another reason to keep using a DE razor, for me they simply shave better.

Review: Gillette Silver Blue

October 9, 2014

Before trying Gillette Silver Blue, manufactured in
Russia and sold by Gillette, questions naturally arise
in one's mind: Why Silver Blue? Shouldn't it be
Bluish Silver? Or Silvery Blue? Perhaps we'll never
know, but what I do know is this: these are some fine
razor blades.

After spending a week with one of Gillette's other
products, the Mach3, it was great to get back to a
double-edge razor. I missed the weight, the skill, the
balance. The slow methodical work that results in a
great shave. It was a risk trying out an unknown
blade, might have spoiled the fun if it turned out to be
a poor fit for my face.

Luckily, that was not the case. I found myself getting
consistent, close shaves. In fact, very few blades that
I've tried held an edge as well as they did. By the end
of the week, when most blades are showing signs of
struggle, the Silver Blues still felt sharp and
smooth. Very few blades shaved as close, very few
gave so little irritation, and even less had both.

The only complaint I have about the blades isn't
related to the shave at all. Depending on how a brand
packages their razors, they can come out of the paper
with little dollops of glue on the blade. Sometimes
it's dry, other times sticky. In the case of the Silver
Blues it was stickier than usual, which by the end of
the week made for a mess to clean up.

But really those were small potatoes compared to the great experience they provided. They were a joy to use and gave some of the best shaves I've had since switching to a DE razor. The only blade that in my mind currently stands with them are Feathers, which means that at some point I'll probably need to do a head to head comparison. I don't know that I'll give them the top spot just yet, but they are a fierce competitor.

In short, the Silver Blues are some of the best razor blades I've used. They are sharp and slick. I highly recommend them.

Dollar Shave Club Review - The Whole Kit and Caboodle

October 20, 2014

Journalistic integrity requires a writer to say when they are reviewing a product whether they paid for it or it was given to them for review, that way people are aware whether there has been inducement.

Or something like that, I think. I'm not a journalist, and I have no idea what their ethical standards happen to be. I just write, and if companies want to send me stuff then so be it. Which Dollar Shave Club (DSC) did, and so here's my unvarnished opinion on it:

If I didn't already own a double-edge (DE) razor I would seriously consider getting a subscription.

To get the full experience I decided to go all in: DSC shaving butter, razors, and after shave moisturizer (I'll review the shave butter and moisturizer as part of DE shaving next week). While the heart of the DSC marketing strategy is selling razor cartridges for cheaper than what you can get Gillette or Schick in stores, and the razor is the most important part of a shave, I'd heard good things about the shave butter and I wanted to judge it with all factors leaning in it's favor (I went into it skeptical, and I didn't want any bias against cartridge razors to tip things too much).

The razor itself seems to be solidly built, perhaps more so than a Mach3. The weight feels heavier, and the cartridge seems to fit more securely to the handle, giving it an overall feel of being higher quality. Where it falls short is the ergonomic design they have tried to put into it, while it works well for shaving downward if you try to hold the razor to shave across the grain or against the grain the ergonomic curves made it awkward for me to hold. In that regard the Mach 3, with it's straighter handle, feels better for those passes, though your mileage may vary.

At first I wasn't very impressed with the shave results. I started with a two day growth, and the shave I got was, at best, adequate. Without careful attention it was easy to miss spots, making the shave as long as what it normally takes with a DE razor. It took two to three passes, with, across, and against the grain, to get a close shave, which sort of seems to defeat the point of a multi-blade razor. Additionally, the size of the four razor head made it difficult to get right under my nose, and there's no single blade trimmer on it. However after a couple days of shaving I found the results improving noticeably, which might mean that some of the above problems were user related. Within a few days I was getting consistently good shaves, which while not as close as what a DE razor offers were still rather good.

The shave butter itself seems similar to the shaving cream sold by Trader Joe's, which worried me a bit at first because when I've tried the Trader Joe stuff it (though working well shave wise) had a tendency to

clog up my razor. Either the two products are
different or I just didn't notice it this time, because I
had no clogging problems with the shave
butter. With some hot water it washed out well, and I
found that a single application of shave butter was
often enough for two or three passes.

The moisturizer took some getting used to. I've never
used a lotion or moisturizer consistently, and I found
the instructions to apply liberally to have been
misleading: don't. A little bit goes a long way, and
after using the shave butter it generally took a few
moments to really soak in. My face would feel slick,
almost oily for several hours afterward, and if I
worked out within a few hours of applying the sweat
would seem to mix with whatever the moisturizer
had left to make it feel like it had just been
applied. Perhaps this is a just what having
moisturized skin feels like. If it's not for you, of
course, you could always just use a regular aftershave
and not order it when you get the razor.

The results have been that after a couple days use I
found myself getting good shaves with no
irritation. The skin butter seems to work well with
the razor, the razor seems to shave as well as any
other cartridge blade, and the moisturizer seems to do
it's job of cooling and soothing any potential burn
spots.

However, I don't see myself signing up for it. If I
were still using a cartridge razor, then this would be
an extremely attractive offer. Cartridges are
extremely expensive, and the idea of having new

razors for dirt cheap along with shaving lather and aftershave stuff shipped right to the door sounds like a heck of a deal. But at the end of the day the shaves, though quite good, were just...dull. Not the razors themselves, mind you, those were quite sharp. Rather the lack of skill involved, the lack of effort required, it made the experience an extremely easy and effective chore, but a chore non-the-less. Within a few days I found myself missing my DE, not simply because of the shave it gives, but because I missed the detail, the effort, and the satisfaction that comes from seeing the fruits of your own labor.

Cartridge razors simply don't offer that, and while DSC gives a good shave it's too simple for my taste. That said, if you're goal is simply to get a close, clean, irritation free shave, then this is right up your ally. It's a solid setup, and the price is hard to argue with. At just a few bucks a month it is considerably higher than a safety razor (DSC advertises on Facebook that its razors cost $4 a month, which can get you half a year or more of safety razor blades), but substantially less than if you bought Gillette cartridges in the same amount. If safety razors aren't for you but you still want to put a hurt on that scruff, then this seems like a good option.

Dollar Shave Club Review - Shave Butter and Moisturizer

October 26, 2014

As I said in my last review, the DSC shave butter and moisturizer did well as part of the complete DSC experience. But it's one thing to keep irritation down when the tool you're using is a cartridge razor, it's nigh impossible to cut yourself with one and if your skin isn't inclined to get sore easily you can shave with just about anything. For years I simply used water.

But the question remained: how would it do under double-edge conditions? A DE razor can give you a closer shave with less irritation than any cartridge...if you use it right. And part of using it right means having a good lather and aftershave to go along with it, or in this case, shave butter and moisturizer. To find out if it would hold up I loaded up a Feather razor blade and gave it a try.

The results were very promising. Throughout the testing I noticed no noticeable razor burn from the shave, and my skin definitely felt good especially with a cold wind that settled in the last few days. Two applications of shave butter was enough to get three passes with the DE, one for with the grain and across the grain, one for against the grain. The shave butter rinsed well out of the blade, and what spots that were missed were likely a result of the user.

But for as well as it worked, there were a few things that have left me ready for a change. First, while it is extremely convenient to just squeeze something out of a tube I miss the enjoyment and ritual (and warmth) that comes from mixing up a warm lather from a block of soap. It's relaxing and refreshing. Second, because the shave butter is almost completely clear it makes it difficult to see where you've shaved and where you haven't. Of course by the end of the shave you should easily see where you still need to shave, but during the initial pass or two when you're trying to reduce rather than remove it can make it difficult to tell what still needs to be done.

A couple things I've noticed about the moisturizer: First, while it soaks in just fine after you put it on I found that it left my face feeling oily for several hours afterward. Or maybe that's just what moisturized skin feels like. It was especially noticeable after exercising, as sweat would seem to draw it out of where it had soaked in. Second, I noticed during the time I was using it an increase of smudges and smears on my cell phone. I think it has been a result of touching my face and picking up some of the lotion residue, then touching the screen. I don't know that's the reason, perhaps I just noticed something that was happening before, but it seemed to be.

Really though these complaints, if they even fall to that level rather than less than enthusiastic noticing, are minor compared to the good results that I have had from using them. If the DSC razors are up your ally, these likely will be too. They'll stay on my shaving counter and I will use them from time to time, but I'm looking forward to getting back to soaps and splashes.

Movember- Why I'm Still Shaving

November 2, 2014

Movember is upon us again, a time when men stop
shaving their mustache in an effort to raise awareness
about men's health issues such as colon cancer (or
simply because they're riding the cultural wave). It's
a worthy cause, but not one I'll be participating in for
a couple reasons.

First, I look awful in a mustache. I shaved a beard
down to one once. My wife took one look and
literally covered her eyes and hid. Actions spoke
louder than words. Jack Kemp once said, "Winning is
like shaving- you do it every day or you wind up
looking like a bum." I'm not sure what I looked like,
but I had to shave it off before she would stop
winching every time she looked at me.

But the larger reason that I'm not shaving is this:
Shaving for me is a manly tradition. A combination
of tools, skill, patience, focus, and practice. I use a
double-edge razor for many reasons, one of which is
that it takes work. Work is good for the mind, body
and soul, and it's something I don't want to go
without.

By all means, grow your beard. I've done so, and I
likely will again. But it makes no sense for me to
deny myself of a manly ritual in an effort to
demonstrate manliness, and in the case of a mustache,

which has the very possible side effect of making me look like some hipster.

That's not how I roll.

Review: Perma-Sharp Super

November 10, 2014

After shaving with the Perma-Sharps for two weeks I'm still not sure how I feel about them, though it's entirely possible that by the time I finish writing this review I'll have talked myself into one opinion or another.

It's an odd blade. The store I bought them from says they are made by Procter & Gamble, but they don't bear the Gillette trade name which P&G owns. They are manufactured in Russia with an English name, which isn't unusual unto itself, except that the package then has what Google translate tells me is Turkish printed right on the front. And when it comes to shaving, it's one of the few blades that have really grown on me.

Most of the time if I'm going to like a blade I can tell pretty quickly. With the Perma-Sharp it was very different. My first shave with it left much to be desired, the next day continued to be unimpressive. But by the third day I found much of what I disliked disappearing. By the fourth day those things weren't even noticeable. By the fifth I had figured I just had a bad start.

Then I changed blades, and it was back to square one. Once again though by the third day or so it was shaving great and I was happy with it.

149

I've had blades that required a bit of time to break in before, I even wrote a blog post about it. But I've never had one with such a steep and noticeable curve. The first couple shaves the blade felt rough, uneven, pulling and tugging when it should be cleanly cutting. But after a shave or two this had vanished, replaced by a reliable, sharp, consistent blade. In fact, by the end of the week I hadn't noticed a decline in sharpness or shave quality. It was living up to its name.

Hence my uncertainty about it. On one hand, for the first shave or two I simply didn't enjoy it. By about Tuesday it was doing well, and it was a pleasure the rest of the week.

Next time I use them I'm going to try out a trick I've heard about, that if you run an overly aggressive razor through a cork that it will even out the edge and give a more comfortable shave. Perhaps that will do the trick. For now, when I get critical about it I remember how smooth and sharp it felt during a time of the week that many razors struggle, but I can't ignore the rough few days at the beginning.

Review: Col. Conk's Shave Soap- Almond

November 15, 2014

For the last four months my primary shaving soap has been Col. Conk's Almond. I bought it in Wall, SD, at a giant general store/ restaurant/ tourist trap they have there (it's probably half of the entire town), along with a couple other Conk's scents. Every kind they had, in fact, except lime. Because who wants to smell like limes in the morning?

Admittedly, before then I would have also asked "who wants to smell like almonds in the morning," or ever really. But it seemed like a good idea at the time and I'm glad I took the risk because it has been a pleasure to use.

I've used Col. Conk's before, and for all I know this is the exact same stuff except with a different fragrance added. Previously the soap sat as a block of soap on a dish, but with this puck I melted it down into a shave bowl right from the start. My technique was then to go in about ten minutes before I would shave, cover the soap with about a quarter-inch of hot water, then let it sit while I got cleaned up and prepared. Once I was ready to shave I'd drain the water, then use a wet brush to load the softened soap and lather on my face.

It worked like gang busters.

Previously I was getting inconsistent loads which resulted in some thin lathers that weren't always enough to get the job done. Perhaps because I'm now more experienced I've great lathers almost every time, and when the load has been insufficient a couple drops of water on the soap and a quick reload got me into good shape. It does seem to have resulted in the soap not lasting as long as the previous puck of Conk's I used, but that might be a result of me not lathering properly previously. Even if this goes though more soap than necessary, when it's still lasting four months I'm not feeling too bad.

The soap provided great protection, and a refreshing scent that made for an enjoyable shave. The scent started extremely strong, dropping off quickly over a couple weeks time, however despite the decline it remained present when lathering up until the last several weeks. I still catch it from time to time, but I think it might be that it's just on its last leg.

I haven't been using it exclusively. I've also been using Proraso, Dollar Shave Club Shave Butter, and Barbasol. But Conk's has been my favorite, hands down. It smells great, feels great, and works great. I've got two more pucks to go through, one Bayrum and the other Amber, and when I'm done I may just find myself stocking back up on Almond. I've highly enjoyed it.

Review: Wilkinson Sword

November 21, 2014

Why shave with a knife, when you can shave with a sword?

Wilkinson Sword is one of the biggest shaving companies in the world, but you probably know them by another name: Schick. For reasons that I'm sure make sense to someone, Wikipedia says company is marketed as Schick in North America, Australia, Asia, and Russia, and Wilkinson Sword everywhere else. As I have been unable to find any Schick labeled double-edge razors, it would seem that portion of their market is handled exclusively through the Sword portion.

But I digress.

The Sword has been a good razor blade. I encountered some roughness on the first shave or two, but once broken in it gave a decent shave through the rest of the week. I did notice is that they seemed harder to clean off, the soap and hair seemed to want to stick to the blade a bit, and the first shave almost felt dull compared to what they did after a day or two of use. But the shaves were close, even, and consistent throughout the week.

And...average. While it was a good shave, I really can't think of any thing that stands out about them except that few other razors had as little irritation as it did. But since very few double-edge razors give me significant irritation, it's really a marginal benefit.

They're good blades, I'll give them that. But while there wasn't anything really bad about them, I don't find myself having a desire to keep using them.

A Brief and Questionably Accurate Explanation of Carbon and Stainless Steel Razor Blades

December 1, 2014

You have probably never asked yourself whether you use a carbon or stainless steel razor blade (perhaps because normality abounds in your life). It's not a question that gets asked often, and because nearly all razor blades are made out of stainless steel, whether in a cartridge or double-edge, it's a question with an easy answer. But that wasn't always the case.

The exact history is somewhat murky, but here is what I've been able to learn...

When Gillette introduced the double-edge safety razor in 1904 all blades were made out of carbon steel, and this continued for almost 60 years. Using carbon steel created a significant problem though: because of the water involved in shaving there was significant risk that a blade would become rusty even over just a few days use, requiring either close care or frequent replacement.

To combat this Gillette turned to metallurgists to do science-y things. By 1945 they began experimenting with coating the blades with a thin layer of other material to protect them, and in short order they turned to polytetraflouroethylne (PTFE), better known as Teflon. They discovered that they could create a blade which, though initially slightly inferior than an untreated razor, would break in after a shave or two and then provide a sharper, longer lasting edge (for those of you interested in details of this, which go over my head, check out the above link).

This all came to a head in the 1960's, when stainless steel was introduced. Depending on who you ask it was either Gillette or Wilkinson Sword who was the first to bring stainless steel to market, but by the mid-sixties it was conquering the market. The blades, often coated with PTFE as well, would last far longer than carbon steel resulting in much reduced need to purchase replacements. With patents expiring, fierce competition, and emerging products that required less purchases, it is little surprise that within a decade of stainless steel blades hitting the market that Gillette introduced the first cartridge razor blade, setting the course of modern shaving.

So if during that brief window stainless steel so thoroughly stomped on carbon steel, why use them? Stainless is so preferred, after all, that there are only a handful of brands that use carbon and most of these can be tough to come by (and only one that I know of that doesn't use PTFE, a Treet brand nicknamed "black beauty").

The edge. Carbon steel hasn't completely died off because they offer a great edge. There is some debate over whether stainless steel or carbon steel blades are harder, and which one degrades faster, but most seem to agree that carbon steel offers an unusually sharp edge at the very beginning. While some say that the carbon steel dulls faster, others contend that the material allows for the edge to be kept far longer than with stainless, and even stropped for longer use.

At the same time, while carbon steel razors are comparable to stainless steel blades, their relative price has plummeted over the decades. Even if the blades are not cared for closely and require more frequent replacement, the cost is still so low that it is not economically prohibitive. If you use twice as many blades, replacing them more frequently, the cost difference amounts to just a few dollars a year (if that). The economic incentive of stainless, while still there, has been greatly reduced.

While the benefits of the two can be debated, what can't be dismissed is that stainless steel remains the dominant force on the market. It is ironic that a method which draws so heavily on heritage and use of techniques and designs that have been around for a century primarily uses blades that appeared within the last few decades.

But if you want to try the type of razor blade that safety razors were originally built for you've still got options. Not many, but they're out there.

Review: Treet Dura Sharp

December 5, 2014

The most significant difference between modern safety razors and wet shaving compared with how it was done a century ago is that today almost all razor blades are made out of stainless steel, while prior to the 1960s razor blades were made out of carbon steel. Carbon steel rusts easier, and so with the introduction of stainless steel carbon steel, despite many feeling carbon held a superior edge, it was almost completely abandoned.

Almost.

Treet Dura Sharp is one of the few razor blades still on the market that's made out of carbon steel. Manufactured in Pakistan, it is coated in PTFE (Teflon) which provides some protection against rusting while also giving a sharper, longer edge over just carbon. Having never used a carbon blade before I was curious how well it would work. I'm sold.

I don't know if the razor is quite as sharp as a Feather, nor quite as smooth as the Gillette Silver Blues. But they have been some of the most enjoyable blades I've shaved with, and they are in serious competition with those two for the spot of my favorite blade. They feel sharp, gave a close shave with no irritation, nicks or bleeding, and they have a satisfying feel (and sound) as they cut through the stubble. The result was a good shave throughout the week, though they had begun to lose some sharpness by the fifth shave or so, and a blade that even if not the best in one category did everything well in an enjoyable, balanced package.

The drawback here, of course, is that since it is carbon steel whether it would rust. I had heard a few different methods of preventing it, with the two leading methods being simply making sure it was well dried (I did this by shaking and blowing it out), or by dipping it at the end of the shave in some rubbing alcohol and letting it air dry (the idea being that the alcohol will displace water, and then dry faster).

I tried both methods, here are the results:

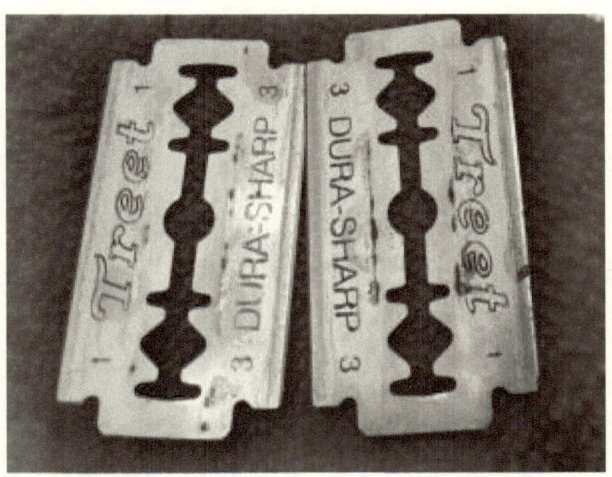

After one week use, alcohol dipped on the left and simply dried on the right. The spot on the blade edge either was fluff or appeared during the week since the blade was used.

Rusting was minimal in both cases, confined to where the razor head clamps down on the blade. There is slightly less rust using the alcohol dip, though during the alcohol week I found myself enjoying how the blade aged through use somewhat less than without. If any actual difference occurred, then to me it would seem that the blade ages better naturally rather than trying to extend its life.

The rusting though is so slight that unless you intend on using the blade longer than a week there seems little cause for concern. They are cheap enough that even if you only shave one or twice a week and can extend the calendar day use of a blade longer than a week then if rusting is a problem you could replace it more often without much added cost. For me though it's not a problem, I change blades every week and if it can survive in Virginia then I suspect it can survive most places.

I highly recommend this blade. Having tried a fair number at this point, it is easily in my top three and might even be my favorite. It's sharp, smooth, and enjoyable. With ten blades a pack I'm looking forward to eight more weeks of fantastic shaves.

Oh Christmas Beard, Oh Christmas Beard...

January 1, 2015

My wife jokes that when we were first dating and first married she could tell the day of the week by my beard, I'd shave on Sunday for church and then grew it through the week. While she has been nothing but supportive of this bizarre shaving endeavor, she has at times expressed an interest in me growing something again. For the Christmas vacation I decided to give her what she wanted and on the 19th the beard began its return.

But that doesn't mean I've stopped shaving completely, and for the last two weeks I've been working to keep my face from being an uncultivated wild. For the first week or so, due to us traveling for the holidays, I pulled out the Dollar Shave Club razor they sent me a couple months back.

It was terrible, and here's why:

When I was a kid my dad wisely made me mow the lawn on Saturday. He also wanted me to edge the lawn, but I would usually just go over it with the mower and figure it was good (eventually we worked out a compromise where I would mow and he would edge).

Trying to use the DSC razor to fine trim a beard was like trying to use the mower to edge the lawn, it's just not the right tool for the job. The razor is great for cutting down lots of hair quickly and without hassle, much like a lawn mower. But the cartridge head is large, the razor is bulky for anything other than simple passes, and the cutting edge is shrouded for safety's sake so it is hard to see exactly where the shaving begins and ends.

Once we got back I switched to my DE razor, loaded with a Wilkinson Sword blade (which I thought would be good enough, but not so nice that I dislike using it for so small a job). Much, much better. I can see the razor so I can fine tune exactly what is getting shaved, it's easier to maneuver, and since it shaves closer the line is more defined. Excellent.

As I've watched the beard grow slowly back in, and as I find myself increasingly anticipating shaving it off, I've taken the time to reflect: in the last year I've tried six shaving creams, three aftershaves, three razors, and a dozen different razor blades. I've liked most of them to some degree, disliked a few, and really enjoyed a small handful. My top three favorite blades have been Feather, Gillette Silver Blue, and Treet Dura-Sharp, and it's a close call between them for who's in first. So close in fact that I really can't say, I'll have to put them head-to-head.

With the new year having arrived I find myself wondering what the future holds. I don't know that this time next year I'll still be writing about shaving, but then again, I wouldn't have thought a year ago I would now have written over a hundred pages on the subject.

The Great Shave

Several years ago I walked into a small model train shop in Mobile, AL, wherein I found an extraordinary display. Everything was meticulous, an incredible example of time, dedication, and attention detail. I asked the clerk about it, and he told me that it was built by him and another enthusiast. Reflecting on the other guy, he chuckled and remarked, "we were working one day on this, and he was using a jeweler's eyepiece and a dental pick to paint pupils on a model duck. He suddenly stopped, set down his tools, looked at me and said, 'what on earth am I doing?' He got up, waked out, and he never came back."

Hobbies have a way of swallowing your time, what begins as a distraction becomes an interest, an interest becomes a routine, and soon enough you find yourself immersed. So found I at the end of last year, when Christmas afforded me a welcome opportunity to step away for a while and grow a beard.

I make no claim to being the world's best beard grower, but by five weeks it was thick enough to fairly claim that I was no longer "growing" a beard, but rather "had" one. Long enough to be soft, as well as troublesome while eating. School returned and I found myself rested, not just from my work but from my hobbies. I was ready to get back into the routine. A wise and prudent man probably would have used some clippers to trim things down to stubble length, then clean it up with normal shaving.

I am not that man.

Instead, I made ready to do battle on a scale never before attempted...by me. I chose my tools carefully: For lather, I went with Proraso green. It's a good, thick lather, and I hoped that the menthol would help alleviate any razor burn that the heavy work might cause. For a blade I picked Treet Dura-Sharp. Carbon steel and one of my favorites, it holds a strong, sharp edge. It would only need to last one shave, but it would be a big one.

With that as a start I softened things with warm water, then lathered up. I don't know that I've ever used more lather at once than I did then, working it from multiple angles to make sure it didn't just gather on the outside but worked down to the skin. Once ready, with razor in hand, I went to work.

The biggest problem became rapidly apparent: there was so much hair that the razor quickly gummed up. Hot water did the trick for that, by breaking down the soap binding the stubble together I was able to clean out the razor with a little effort but each pass quickly made a new mess. With the deftness and subtle of a Cub Scout with a hatchet, I hacked away.

It took four passes to get things set right. Two with the grain, the first to get to clear the hair, the second to clear the stubble. Once across the grain, and a final pass with the grain to get things nice and smooth. To wrap things up I first used a spice aftershave to tighten the skin, then a splash of Lucky Tiger face tonic to cool things off.

Remarkably, irritation was at most mild, and only noticeable when I'd rub a certain part of my neck. The beard was gone (to some disappointment to my wife), and I was ready to get back in the grove. I've grown to love my shaving routine, and I'm excited to have it back.

For now.

About the Author

Blake Roberts was born and raised in Mesa, AZ.
After serving as a missionary for The Church of Jesus
Christ of Latter-Day Saints he graduated from
Brigham Young University-Idaho with a degree in
Political Science.

He now resides in Northern Virginia with his wife
Amanda, and their dog Malcolm, where he is a
student at American University's Washington College
of Law and at the American University School of
Public Policy. He blogs about shaving at:
www.amanoverbored.wordpress.com

This is his first accidental book.

www.ingramcontent.com/pod-product-compliance
Lightning Source LLC
Chambersburg PA
CBHW050447290526
45786CB00006B/2196

* 9 7 8 1 5 0 8 8 2 0 3 0 7 *